Professor Felice Jacka is the director of the Food & Mood Centre at Deakin University in Australia. She is the founder and president of the International Society for Nutritional Psychiatry Research and immediate past president of the Australian Alliance for the Prevention of Mental Disorders. She holds Honorary Principal Research Fellow appointments at the Centre for Adolescent Health, Murdoch Children's Research Centre, and the Black Dog Institute. Professor Jacka has pioneered a highly innovative program of research that examines how individuals' diets and other lifestyle behaviours, interact with the risk for mental health problems. Her current research focuses closely on the links between diet, gut health and mental and brain health. This work is being carried out with the ultimate goal of developing new, evidence-based prevention and treatment strategies for mental disorders. She has published more than 150 peer-reviewed scientific papers, the majority in high-impact journals in the mental health field including the *American Journal of Psychiatry*, *World Psychiatry*, *BMC Medicine* and *Lancet Psychiatry*. She is listed in the top ten most highly cited researchers in mood disorders in Australia (Scopus).

'Felice Jacka has written the most authoritative book for the lay-public about the relationship between diet and mental health. Informative and fun to read, it discusses the emerging close relationship between food and brain function in health and in several brain disorders, including depression, anxiety, and Alzheimer's disease. For anybody who enjoys delicious food and is interested in the health of their brain, this is a must-read book!'

Prof Emeran Mayer

'*Brain Changer* is a provocative, accessible and personal journey into why the food we eat may be the best medicine for our brain health. Jacka is leading the way in providing evidence-based approaches that are rooted in cutting-edge science to transform how we think about mental health.'

Prof John Cryan

'When Felice approached me to analyse the diet and mental health data we had on thousands of adolescents in four countries, I said "Go ahead, but I doubt if you will find anything because these are just normal kids and our dietary data are not very comprehensive". She did go ahead and she found the strong associations she predicted and now I am a strong advocate of her key message – what you eat substantially affects your mental health. This evidence is a game-changer.'

Prof Boyd Swinburn

'A fascinating, thoughtful and evidence-based journey into the cutting-edge field of food and the brain – from a brilliant and respected science leader.'

Dr Sandro Demaio

Brain Changer

PROFESSOR FELICE JACKA

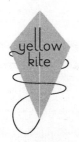

yellow
kite

10% of the author's proceeds will go towards research at the Food & Mood Centre.

First published in 2019 by Macmillan by Pan Macmillan Australia Pty Ltd

First published in Great Britain in 2019 by Yellow Kite
An imprint of Hodder & Stoughton
An Hachette UK company

2

For my very precious mum, Irene (Rene) Jacka,
who always dreamed of writing a book.
1920–2018

Contents

Introduction

I've always been interested in the impact of food on health. I grew up in an unconventional family of naturopaths, where our family dogma was very firmly rooted in the idea that what we put in our mouths formed the foundation of all our bodily processes and, ultimately, our health. That made all sorts of sense to me, although it had to be said that my dear old mum – born in 1920 – was no cook. To be honest, I don't know how she could have made vegetables less tasty. She would boil them until they were a sludgy heap on the bottom of the saucepan and then serve them with no sauces or flavourings. No wonder I grew up not liking vegetables!

Once I left home and started preparing food for myself, my relationship with vegetables changed and I started to appreciate their value as the foundation of every meal. Preparing a large dish of roasted sweet potatoes, tomatoes, zucchini, eggplant and all the other myriad vegetables that make up my family's daily diet, gives me a joy and satisfaction that goes beyond the direct impact of these foods on my health. In so many ways, I truly *love* food – by which I mean *real* food, not manufactured food products – and food has now become the focus of my life's work.

Although I spent my twenties at art school, with no thoughts of science or research, by my thirties I had decided to go back to university to study psychology. A very important reason for this was my personal experience with anxiety and depression. After developing what I now recognise as an anxiety disorder when I was a child – which is not uncommon – by the time I was entering adolescence I had developed quite a severe panic disorder and started to experience regular bouts of depression. This, unfortunately, is also a very common experience for many people. From my late twenties, however, by focusing on exercise, diet and sleep, I had started to recover and stay well. This was my trigger for going back to study. As I progressed through my degree (slowly, due to two small daughters who took up a lot of my time) I began to recognise the interest I had in the brain and the biological aspects of mental health. I also started to become very interested in the idea of research rather than counselling.

By the time I was halfway through my degree I had started to do some interning work in a psychiatry research unit, headed by a wonderful psychiatrist and researcher, Professor Michael Berk. I had found my place, and I thrived in the new world of data and research that started to open up before me. As I studied and learned, I became more and more interested in mental health and the factors that influence whether or not someone will develop depression or anxiety; these are called the 'common mental disorders' for a very good reason.

But I also became increasingly bemused as I realised how different the world of psychiatry and mental health research was from research focused on physical health. This was due to a lack of scientific data concerning the possible role of diet and nutrition in mental health, thanks to an apparent lack of interest in the topic among mental health researchers. In fact, many seemed to have a disdain for the idea that diet might be of relevance to mental health. Suggesting that what we eat might influence how we feel was to many the domain of hippie-trippy, non-evidence-based belief rather than real medicine. And that came right back around to the very good reason that there simply wasn't much in the way of scientific evidence linking food and mood. There was also a lot of misinformation, often propagated by 'alternative' health practitioners, which had further tarnished the reputation of the topic within the research and clinical community.

Given my love of food and my firm belief that what we put in our mouths several times a day is the foundation for every aspect of our health, I decided that I wanted to change the status quo and generate quality information from rigorous science. And so I set out on a journey of research discovery. I began my PhD in 2005, examining the association between women's diets and their mental health, with a focus on the common mental disorders – depression and anxiety. What I found was truly intriguing and set the scene for a whole journey of exploration that has now – more than ten years later – begun to change the way we think about mental and brain health.

This book tells the story of that journey and explains how and why we should consider our food as the basis of our mental and brain health throughout our lives. It also highlights practical things we can do to help prevent mental health problems in the first place, as well as strategies for treating these problems if they do arise. I hope this book provides tools that allow you and your loved ones to optimise your mental and brain health at every stage of life.

PART 1
DIET AND GOOD MENTAL HEALTH

1

Two modern challenges: diet and mental health

It's easy to assume that our modern diet is better than those of hundreds of years ago or even Victorian times, but that, unfortunately, is not the case.

The mid-Victorians, food environments and health

In the United Kingdom in the mid-1800s there was a rare period of unusual good health. Despite the issues with hygiene, infectious diseases and poverty that affected people in urban areas such as London (advances in hygiene and schemes to ensure clean air and water did not start to make an impact on health outcomes until the 1870s), the life expectancy for those who made it to the age of five was as good as or better than it is now in the 21st century. Amazingly, rates of degenerative diseases, such as stroke and cancer, were only 10 per cent of what they are in the

United Kingdom today. And while death from heart disease was not uncommon, it was generally as a result of contracting rheumatic fever, an infectious disease. Overweight and obesity were rare.

Why was this?

Researchers have identified that the main reason for the general public's rude good health during this time was their average diet. The particular political climate of the time meant that politicians had to ensure everybody, even the less well-off, could access and afford fresh meat, vegetables and fruit. Plant foods such as onions, watercress, Jerusalem artichokes, carrots, turnips, broccoli and peas were cheap and easy to access. In fact, many people grew their own vegetables. Apples, cherries, gooseberries and plums were all part of regular diets. Dried beans were very often used as the basis of meals, and people snacked on hazelnuts, walnuts and chestnuts. Almonds and brazil nuts were imported and considered a 'treat' (a stark contrast to our modern-day ice cream, cakes and sweets). Fresh fish and shellfish were also a normal part of people's diets. Red meat was less common because of the cost, but all parts of the animals, such as brains, hearts, liver and kidneys, were eaten and these parts contain many valuable nutrients. Many people kept hens, so eggs were also a part of most people's diets. Bread was eaten in large quantities and made from lightly milled grains that retained their outer husks, full of fibre and nutrients. Finally, although beer was commonly consumed, its alcohol content was far lower than that of modern beers, and other forms of alcohol were less commonly consumed. Of course, pretty much all foods were what we would now consider 'organic', meaning that the population was not exposed to the wide range of chemicals used in industrial farming today.

Most of the jobs, paid and unpaid, of that period also involved quite a lot of physical labour, including the effort spent getting to and from work. This level of energy expenditure meant that calorie intakes – on average – were roughly twice what they are today. In fact, people ate eight to ten portions of fruit and vegetables per day. This meant that nutrient and fibre intake was also much higher, by default. At the same time, salt and sugar intakes were far lower, as these were not commonly added to foods. And the calorie content of foods was much lower.

Unfortunately, this period of excellent nutrition and resulting good health did not last long. Soon imported wheat from North America, as well as new milling techniques, made white flour and bread cheaper and more popular than the traditional varieties. Imported tinned meats, which were very fatty and full of salt, also became cheaper and commonly eaten. Manufactured sweets, condensed milk and tinned fruit with syrup also became widely available, increasing the amount of sugar in people's diets. This extra sugar had such a rapid and detrimental impact on dental health that by 1900 it was noted that many people could no longer chew meat, vegetables, fruits and nuts because of the condition of their teeth!

The state of the nation's health went down so rapidly due to changes in the food supply, as well as new access to manufactured cigarettes and cheap alcohol, that by 1900 fully half of the young men volunteering to fight in the Boer War were rejected because they were so undernourished and weak. During the previous decades, the average worker was very strong, able to 'routinely shovel up to 20 tons of earth per day from below their feet to above their heads'. Between 1880 and 1900, however, these profound changes in nutrition, as well as low access to sunlight and vitamin D among urban dwellers, led to widespread weakness and stunting. As a result, the army had to lower the height requirement for young recruits from five feet six inches to five feet three inches to compensate. This change happened in only two decades.

British officers, who could still afford fresh food and ate less of the tinned and newly processed foods, didn't experience such malnutrition and stunting.

This is a perfect, if sobering, illustration of the enormous impact our food environment can have on population health.

The way we live now

Childhood obesity in the United States has tripled since the 1970s, and today nearly 60 per cent of America's children will be obese by the age of 35. That's not overweight, that's obese. One of my close colleagues here in Australia leads a large research program trying to work out the best ways to prevent obesity in children. They're finding that 40 per cent or more of primary school-aged children in some regional areas are already overweight or obese. Of course, once people are overweight or obese it's very hard to reverse, and this means more and more adults in the same state.

At this moment, roughly two-thirds of American adults are overweight or obese, and the rates are pretty much the same in other Western countries such as Australia and the United Kingdom. In 2007–08, 33.7 per cent of American adults were obese and 5.7 per cent were severely obese – which was bad enough. By 2015–16, however, that had risen to nearly 40 per cent obese and nearly 8 per cent severely obese. It is expected that by 2030, only a few years away, *nearly half* of the American population will be obese. In the United States today, nearly 60 per cent of the population's average calorie intake comes from ultra-processed foods. In Australia it's a bit less – 35 per cent (40 per cent among children and adolescents) – but we're heading in the same direction. This is despite very extensive efforts over many years to educate the public about the dangers of unhealthy eating.

What has happened in the West is now being mirrored in Indonesia, Brazil, China, India and even the poorest countries in Africa. When Mexico opened its trade borders in the 1980s, resulting in a complete transformation of its food environment from traditional diets to Western, industrialised 'foods', obesity rates rose from 7 per cent in 1980 to more than 30 per cent today. Type 2 diabetes is now the leading killer in Mexico, accounting for roughly 80,000 deaths per year. These changes across the world have happened staggeringly and distressingly quickly.

If you live in a Western country, and increasingly if you live in a non-Western country, consider for a moment what you see when you walk into a petrol station to pay for your fuel. Is it wall-to-wall soft drinks? Packaged crisps, chocolates and sweets? Pies, hot dogs and sugary pastries? What about when you walk down the main street – what are most of the food shops selling? Fried chicken and hamburgers? Doughnuts and cakes? Pretzels and greasy meat kebabs? And consider when you attend a hospital, community centre or, in some countries, even a school: are there vending machines full of soft drinks and packaged junk foods? Cafeterias selling mostly cakes, sweet muffins, chips, doughnuts, chocolate and flavoured drinks?

This is the world as most of us now know it, and it has become normal. Public health experts call this the 'obesogenic environment' and note that these sorts of food products (I don't really consider them actual foods) are now the cheapest options for eating, and the most accessible, socially acceptable and heavily advertised.

This has not always been the case, of course. When I was a child in the 1970s (bearing in the mind that my family were more health conscious than most), cakes, chips, sweets and soft drinks were something I had if I went to a birthday party. Fish and chips were an occasional Friday night treat. Portion sizes were smaller. Most people consumed a 'meat and three veg' evening meal, and fruit or a sandwich was a standard snack. You would have to go to a speciality shop, such as a bakery, to buy a cake, pie or doughnut, or make it yourself. Fizzy drinks were treats, and water or milk were the main drinks on offer for us children.

Now, in contrast, think about the young people in your lives today. My husband is a schoolteacher and I work in an area with many secondary schools. What I see as I go to work is teenagers eating pastries, fried foods and thickshakes on their way to school. I see them gather in fast-food outlets after school, eating hamburgers and ice creams and drinking fizzy drinks. I also know that many of them have eaten foods such as white-bread sandwiches with chocolate filling, pizzas, pies and packaged snacks while they were at school. And a large number of them will go home to snack on chips, biscuits and sugary drinks both before and after their dinner. And many of these young people don't look like I or my friends did when we were in high school – they're several sizes larger. Unsurprisingly. (Although even the ones who aren't overweight or obese may still be eating a terrible diet. Youth, exercise and genes can all mean that some young people avoid weight gain even when their diet is poor – but it doesn't mean that it's not affecting their short- and long-term health. We'll talk more about that later.)

Our modern food environment

The rise of the industrial and globalised food industry, which recognised more than 100 years ago that food products with a long shelf life could be produced very cheaply and that people would flock to buy them for their taste and convenience, has meant that our global food environment has changed profoundly. And this new normal has had a devastating impact on our health.

It wasn't so long ago that a *lack* of food was generally understood to be a leading cause of premature death across the world, closely followed by infectious diseases such as malaria and HIV, as well as common childhood killers such as diarrhoeal infections. Of course, these still account for shortened lifespan in many parts of the world, and rear their heads for periods of time in discrete geographical locations (such as during famine and war).

Almost unbelievably, given the rise of large-scale agriculture and our subsequent increased access to food, *poor diet is now the leading risk factor for early death in developed countries and number two worldwide.* Across the entire globe in 2016, the number-one risk factor for death in men and the second leading risk factor for death in women was a diet low in fruits, vegetables, whole grains, nuts and seeds, fibre and good-quality fats from fish and plants, and/or a diet high in processed meats, salt and sugar-sweetened beverages. Such diets accounted for nearly a fifth of all male deaths.

Unhealthy diet leads to early death by increasing the risk of non-infectious illnesses such as heart disease, hypertension (high blood pressure), stroke, high blood glucose and type 2 diabetes, many forms of cancer and, of course, overweight and obesity. In fact, across the world, being overweight now kills more people than being underweight, even in many countries where undernutrition has historically been a very important cause of death.

In 2011 the World Health Organization (WHO) called an emergency meeting in New York to work out what to do about the diet-related chronic illnesses that are challenging communities and governments everywhere. The head of WHO, Dr Margaret Chan, estimated that by 2030 the cost of diet-related disease to the global economy was likely to be at least US$30 trillion, noting that no economy in the world was rich enough to bear this cost. She also stressed, very clearly, that the *only* way to address this problem was for the leaders of governments to take firm action against the multinational corporations profiting enormously from the changes to the world's dietary habits.

Did anything change? Nope, not so far. Has the obesity/chronic disease epidemic started to abate? No, not a bit. Are these food products still widely available, cheap, and heavily promoted? You bet. Have there been restrictions on their availability or marketing? Not much so far.

This makes me really cross. In fact, it's *the* main issue that motivates me to get out of bed every day to do my work.

But WHO and similar organisations are omitting one extremely important consideration when they calculate the cost of poor diets to global health: it's not only our physical health but also our mental and brain health that are affected. This very important fact is the focus of this book.

The Global Burden of Disease study

One of the main reasons we know about the impact of poor diet on disease and death is a very large and comprehensive research program called the Global Burden of Disease (GBD) study, which involves more than 1800 researchers in more than 180 countries across the world. The GBD team systematically gathers evidence on the prevalence of diseases, and their causes and consequences (illness and death), across all 21 regions of the planet. The research is funded by the Bill and Melinda Gates Foundation and the results are regularly published in the leading medical journal, *The Lancet*. The study tells us many important things about how the health of the world's population is changing: some of the news is pretty good and other news is not so good.

For example, while life expectancy increased in most countries between 2005 and 2015, and death from most types of cancer decreased due to better prevention and treatment, total deaths from Alzheimer's disease and other dementias increased by almost 40 per cent. This is largely due to population growth and the increasing age of the population in many countries. While many nations in sub-Saharan Africa experienced improvements in life expectancy as deaths from HIV/AIDs and malaria decreased, other parts of the world have actually seen decreases in life expectancy due to war (for example in Syria) and sustained levels of mortality from interpersonal violence (such as gun-related deaths in the United States). Heart disease and stroke remain the leading causes of death globally, while lung cancer also remains a major killer, despite large reductions in the number of smokers in many countries.

Clearly, the drivers for many of the risk factors for death are highly diverse. Poverty, war, famine and lack of access to health care remain enormous challenges for many countries, and have highly complex and historically intractable causes.

On the other hand, poor diet has one leading cause globally. And while addressing this cause also presents many challenges, there is one main, clear target: the global industrial food industry. Big Food. This potentially makes things simpler. We'll talk more about this later, but first let's have a look at mental and brain health.

Where do mental disorders fit in?

The GBD study doesn't just examine and document causes of death, it also covers 'disability', which measures the loss of health (but not death) associated with having a particular illness. When the information from around the globe is considered through this lens, the leading causes of disability are actually not illnesses in the traditional sense, but what are collectively called mental and substance use disorders. These include what we call the common mental disorders – depression and anxiety disorders (including major depressive disorder, panic disorder, post-traumatic stress disorder, obsessive-compulsive disorder, social phobias and generalised anxiety disorder); the less common illnesses, such as schizophrenia and bipolar disorder; and drug and alcohol disorders. They also include eating disorders, such as anorexia and bulimia; childhood behavioural disorders (attention deficit hyperactivity disorder, or ADHD); and what are called pervasive developmental disorders, such as autism and Asperger's syndrome.

Of all of these, major depressive disorder – what we commonly just call depression – is by far the main contributor, representing more than 40 per cent of the burden of these disorders as a group. Anxiety disorders make up the next largest piece of the pie. In fact, depression consistently features as one of the top-five leading causes of disability across the planet. Given the impact of this disorder on the health and wellbeing of people throughout the world, and the fact that the bulk of the evidence regarding the relationship between diet and mental health comes from depression studies, let's consider this disorder in a bit more detail.

Like many teenagers, I suffered from depression and anxiety during my adolescence. For many young people, these common mental disorders, depression in particular, first rear their ugly heads around puberty. Large biological changes, along with big life changes, make this period one of particular risk for mental health problems. In fact, half of all mental disorders first manifest before the age of fourteen. For many people, these go on to become recurrent and sometimes chronic conditions. While the good news is that these illnesses disappear for good for many sufferers by their mid-twenties, it remains an unfortunate fact that depression is exceedingly common in adolescents.

Here in Australia, a recent large-scale survey reporting on the mental health of children and adolescents aged between four and 17 highlighted just how common these disorders are in this age group: nearly one in five girls aged 16–17 were found to meet the criteria for clinical depression, while approximately one in ten young people indicated that they had engaged in self-harming behaviour in the past year. Anxiety disorders, which have a very early age of onset, were also common, affecting nearly 7 per cent of the survey participants in the previous 12 months.

The risk factors for depression and other mental illnesses

One of the key findings from this large survey is that coming from a family with a low income and/or low education level is a particular risk factor for mental health problems. In fact, in this study, children and adolescents from families in the lowest income bracket were twice as likely to have a mental disorder than those in the highest income bracket. These findings echo what we see in studies from across the globe: poverty and social and economic disadvantage profoundly influence the risk of mental health problems in both young people and adults. Other risk factors are genetics – people with a family history of mental health problems, including depression, are at greater risk of developing these disorders than those with no such family history – as well as early life trauma and abuse and life stresses. These factors are all linked to an increased risk of lifelong mental health problems.

One very notable thing about these risk factors is, to my mind, just how difficult they are to change. Certainly, we can't change our genes, although we may be able to influence what they do (more about this later) and, of course, poverty and social disadvantage are particularly intractable problems that appear to be quite resistant to intervention (or so politicians would have us believe).

The relative difficulty in changing these risk factors, I believe, is why we lack – to my knowledge anyway – any structured, evidence-based strategies or blueprints for the *prevention* of mental disorders in any country. But if diet were found to be a risk factor for mental disorders, wouldn't this suggest that we could think seriously about prevention? Isn't prevention always better than cure? What if I told you that we now believe, based on good evidence, that diet *is* a modifiable risk factor for mental illness?

This is not to say that it's the *whole* cause of mental illness – given the complexity of risk factors and the way they interact, that would certainly be overselling the case. But if we identify a risk factor for mental disorders that *can* be changed, shouldn't we attempt to do so? Particularly if it's something that affects 100 per cent of the population every single day? A lot of what this book is about has this idea of *prevention* as an underpinning concept.

How depression looks and feels

I always say that depression felt to me like I'd been attacked by a dementor from the Harry Potter books. Dementors suck all the life and joy out of a person and leave their victims devoid of happy feelings and unable to experience pleasure from even joyful events. Of course, everyone experiences illness differently, but this loss of pleasure from even happy events or circumstances is one of the key symptoms of depression. Its official name is anhedonia. Another key symptom required to qualify for depression, either in combination with anhedonia or on its own, is 'depressed mood'.

That is if you're angling for a diagnosis of major depression, which I suspect you're not. Other symptoms can include persistent fatigue, difficulties concentrating and making decisions, unwarranted feelings of guilt and worthlessness, appetite and sleep disturbances, slowness or agitation in bodily movements, and thoughts of death. Some of these symptoms, in combination with either anhedonia and/or depressed mood, need to be present for at least two weeks and cause significant distress or impairments to functioning (in other words, impact on your ability to go to work, look after your family or the like). It's a really horrible illness and I wouldn't wish it on my worst enemy. My early experiences with depression prompted my interest in studying psychology; I wanted to understand what caused this awful illness and what I could do to stop it ever happening again.

How anxiety looks and feels

I'm betting I don't need to tell you this. Almost everyone experiences anxiety at times – it's a normal part of being human. A bit of anxiety can be a useful thing, forcing us to pay attention and take care to avoid danger or problems. But a lot of anxiety can be crippling and have a very big impact on quality of life. There are many different anxiety disorders. One very common one is phobias. Most people don't love spiders, snakes or sharks, but when a fear of these starts to really interfere with their lives, it's classified as a disorder. Similarly, social phobia is very common. People with social phobia feel the eyes of the world upon them. They shrink from social interaction and this can, again, have a big impact on their day-to-day functioning. Generalised anxiety disorder affects many people, making them worry endlessly about almost every little thing. This can be crippling. Then there is post-traumatic stress disorder (PTSD), which can arise after traumatic events of all kinds, and obsessive-compulsive disorder (OCD). PTSD and OCD can be particularly serious and devastating. So can panic disorder, which both I and my eldest daughter suffered from for years. People with anxiety disorders will often avoid social situations or fear leaving the house, which can really impact their quality of life.

If you think you might be suffering from anxiety or depression, as a first step complete the beyondblue checklist on their website – seeking help from your doctor is the next step.

Are mental and brain illnesses on the rise?

Hmm, this is a tricky question. It's exceedingly difficult to measure a slippery illness like depression through time. There are many obstacles to accurately measuring changes in levels of psychological symptoms across different groups of people. Large surveys generally use different assessment measures over different time points, and people's understanding of, and the official criteria for, depression and other mental illnesses change over time. For this reason, there's much debate as to whether mental disorders or psychological distress in the wider population have actually increased – either in adults or young people.

There is, however, some evidence of an increase in common mental disorders and psychological distress from a range of Western countries, including the United States, the United Kingdom, Australia and Taiwan. This seems to be particularly the case among young people. Here in the state of Victoria, a very recent report told us that presentations to emergency departments by children (up to 18 years old) for extreme mental distress and self-harm had increased by roughly 50 per cent over the past ten years or so. So there's some evidence that things are getting worse. Certainly, it suggests that whatever we're doing to address this major cause of suffering and distress in our communities is not working very well.

In contrast, there doesn't seem to be much evidence for increases in the rates of psychotic illnesses, such as schizophrenia, although this illness is more common in urban areas in developed countries. There are, however, some very worrying data on reported increases in neurodevelopmental disorders – particularly autism spectrum disorder (ASD), which has risen in the United States from one case per 25,000 children in the 1950s to one case in every 50 children in 2013. Although some studies and researchers believe that this very large increase in rates of ASD is the result of increased recognition and diagnosis, many studies and researchers believe this to only be part of the reason for the increase. Some speculate on the possible driving role of Western diets and their negative effects on immune function, and highlight the parallel very large increases in allergic disease in children over a similar time period. We'll explore this in coming chapters.

Finally, although it's not officially a mental disorder, it's worth considering dementia, the most common manifestation of which is Alzheimer's disease. Due to advances in medical science, many of us are living longer lives, which means that rates of dementia are definitely increasing, simply because we have more opportunity to develop it. But do we want to? Of course not. So what can we do to reduce our risk of dementia? What can we do to protect our brain health so that we can continue to think, learn and interact, with our on-board computer in good condition, until we leave this world for good? Research tells us that remaining intellectually active (that is reading and learning, playing intellectually challenging games and the like) and having good social support are important protective factors against dementia in old age. But the increasing evidence is strongly pointing to lifestyle behaviours such as diet, exercise and smoking as key factors influencing the risk of poor brain health as we age. Again, these are all modifiable – in other words, we have the opportunity to change them and potentially head off the risk of dementia.

Why we need to act now

Poor diet and mental disorders are the leading health issues of the 21st century, and the two most important factors contributing to death and disability across the globe. Our new knowledge that poor diet and mental and brain health are linked has profound implications for the health of individuals and societies, as well as for the public purse. It also suggests the possibility of being able to reduce the risk of and even *prevent* at least some of the burden of mental disorders, an idea that is yet to be put into action.

The following chapters will describe in greater detail what we know about the link between diet and mental and brain health, and offer suggestions for what we might do to act on this new knowledge. This book will gently take you through the latest research from the important new field of Nutritional Psychiatry, and provide useful insights, suggestions and resources to help you apply this new evidence to your life and improve both your health and that of your family.

Key facts

- Poor diet is now the leading risk factor for death across middle- and high-income countries, and number two worldwide.
- In the United States, nearly 60 per cent of average energy intake comes from ultra-processed food products.

- In Australia, roughly 40 per cent of the calories children and adolescents consume come from ultra-processed junk foods.
- Being overweight now kills more people than being underweight.
- Obesity rates have more than doubled since 1980 and tripled since the 1970s.
- Mental and substance use disorders are the leading cause of disability worldwide.
- Half of all mental disorders start before the age of 14.
- The global economic cost of mental disorders was approximately US$2.5 trillion in 2010, and is expected to rise to almost US$16 trillion over the next two decades.

2

Diet and mental health in adults

People often say to me, 'But surely we've known for a long time that diet affects mental health.' It's a fair enough comment, and I think that many people *perceive* that link between what they eat and how they feel. And we also know that many people with depression try changing their diet in order to try to improve their mood. We knew this even before the research on diet and mental health was done. Consider this story for an example. Tim (not his real name) contacted me after hearing me speak on the radio. This is what he said:

> I have experienced the lows of feeling and functioning at low mental mood and a general lack of *joie de vivre*. As an airline captain, it was affecting me not only in my personal life but my professional life. I had a diet that was high in carbohydrates, sugar, processed food and saturated fats. I'd gained weight since my early twenties and was 30 kilograms heavier.

I felt lethargic almost every day. Mornings were slow and evenings simply a means of getting to bed. I was looking forward at life, thinking that something needed to change.

So what to do?

I switched literally overnight. I adopted a diet of fruit and vegetables and occasionally portions of nuts. This was initially as a juice diet for a period of time. High intake of greens such as kale, spinach and silverbeet, with celery, coriander, mint, parsley, apples, ginger and turmeric. Within 72 hours I had a shift and change in my mental acuity, but my mood was ridiculously buoyant. This has been a constant change measure. Each week and month I continued a return to that young guy I knew in my twenties. I started thinking so much more clearly. I swear my eyesight has improved and that women have become more attractive. Well that's possibly a function of just thinking more clearly. My work is more enjoyable and flows more easily, with fewer apparent challenges or stress. Go figure . . .

I hear and have heard stories like this every week for many years. But in order to convince policymakers (government), doctors and other health professionals to take this topic seriously, we need more than just anecdotes. We need research evidence. And not just any research evidence – it needs to be good-quality research evidence. And until the last few years, such evidence linking diet to mental health has been pretty thin on the ground.

Gathering the scientific evidence

Before 2009 there had been a number of studies – some of them of good quality and many of them not so good – examining the possible links between aspects of our diet, such as fish or folate intake, and the risk of developing disorders such as depression. There were also studies examining the possible usefulness of fish oil or folate supplements for depression and other mental disorders. And there were also a few studies looking at the possible link between the levels of nutrients in our blood and either our risk of developing mental disorders or our response to treatments for them, such as antidepressants. While some of these studies considered each of these factors – dietary intakes, the use of supplements or the levels of nutrients in our blood – as being of some use or relevance to mental health, in various others the quality of the studies was poor, meaning that we couldn't glean much in the way of useful insights from them. But the interest was there from many different researchers, from many different fields of study, around the world.

But the big problem with these studies, whether they were of good quality or poor quality, is that we don't eat just individual nutrients such as folate or foods such as fish; we eat whole diets, where a very large number of different compounds interact in very complex ways to affect our health.

As one example, folate is found in many vegetables, fruits and salads, and low folate intake is associated with depression in many studies across the world. But plant foods, in addition to all the nutritional components they contain, such as folate, minerals, proteins, fatty acids, fibre, carbohydrates and the like, also contain thousands of other bioactive compounds, such as carotenoids (found in orange, red and green leafy vegetables), flavonoids (in tea, grapes, red wine, dark chocolate, citrus fruits and berries), glucosinolates (from cruciferous vegetables, such as brussels sprouts, cabbage and broccoli), phytoestrogens (in soy, grains, nuts and seeds), sterols (in vegetable oils, nuts, cereals and some vegetables) and sulfurous compounds (onions, leeks and garlic).

These all interact in highly complex ways, and we're only starting to understand what they do in the body to affect health.

To put this in real terms, imagine what a day in the diet of a healthy eater – let's call him Bert – might look like. His favourite breakfast might be oats (porridge), cooked with some banana and topped with milk, nuts, seeds and some honey. He might make a large salad to take to work for lunch, combining rocket, spinach, watercress, carrots, fresh beetroot, tomatoes, topping it off with a tin of tuna or maybe some ricotta cheese, dressed with olive oil and balsamic vinegar, and a slice of wholegrain sourdough bread. Afternoon tummy-rumbling might be met with almonds, brazil nuts, walnuts and/or cashews, along with an apple. And then dinner could be a big plate of broccoli, cauliflower, sweet potato mash, some brown rice and a small serve of lean steak, with frozen blueberries and yoghurt for dessert. With a glass of red wine. Or it might be a lentil stew or soup, full of vegetables and wholegrain barley. Throughout the day, Bert could be drinking tea – black and green – as well as a couple of coffees with cow's, soy or almond milk.

The number and diversity of fats, fibres, proteins, carbohydrates, vitamins, minerals, polyphenols and many, many other bioactive parts of foods in this lucky person's diet – not to mention the very complex ways they all interact to affect his health – would not even begin to be captured by measuring and reporting on only one nutrient. This would only give us a very tiny, and probably not very useful, part of the picture.

This was also an issue for nutrition research in general – not just in relation to mental health. So scientists started to develop ways we might measure the whole diet rather than just bits of it.

To do this we use statistics and, while I won't bore you to tears with the details (when my husband Rob can't sleep he's been known to say, 'Tell me about your research, darling'), very simply speaking it involves putting the answers from the dietary questionnaires given to people participating in research studies through a statistical process that allows us to measure 'dietary patterns'. These techniques basically quantify how food habits tend to clump together. For example, if people eat higher quantities of vegetables, they often also eat other healthy foods, such as fruit, fish and whole grains. On the other hand, those that drink soft drinks are often likely to also eat processed foods with added sugars, fats and salt. Although this process is certainly not perfect – as you can imagine, measuring people's diets is very tricky, particularly given how much we like to fool ourselves and others into thinking we're eating better than we really are! – over the past decade or so, this new approach has allowed researchers to examine the links between our overall dietary habits and health. We have also introduced new dietary indices, measuring such things as our adherence to a Mediterranean-style diet, or the Healthy Eating Index, or the Dietary Inflammatory Index, or similar. These are also useful ways to measure overall dietary quality.

As you might guess, the research tells us that habitually following healthy (sometimes called 'prudent' or 'whole foods') dietary patterns that are high in plant foods, such as vegetables, fruits, whole grains, nuts, seeds and legumes, as well as fish and olive oil, is consistently associated with a reduced risk for chronic diseases such as heart disease, high blood pressure, many forms of cancer, type 2 diabetes, overweight and obesity, lung diseases, and even age-related eye conditions. On the other hand, following an unhealthy dietary pattern (often referred to as 'Western') higher in added sugars, fats and salt (along with quite a few nasty additives) is more likely to result in those diseases. Similarly, higher adherence to a Mediterranean-style diet, or the Healthy Eating Index or similar, is consistently associated with better health outcomes. This, of course, has been known for quite a while and is reflected in those large GBD studies I discussed in Chapter 1. But what is new is the evidence linking these dietary patterns to mental and brain health, which is what I want to talk about now.

Where it all began (for me)

As I mentioned in the introduction, when I first fell into psychiatry research I was very interested and somewhat bemused to realise that there wasn't much in the way of research examining the links between diet and mental health. When I first came to work with Professor Michael Berk I was still doing my undergraduate degree in psychology and really didn't know much about the field of psychiatry research (or research in general). Luckily, Michael recognised that I was keen to get my hands on some real data and to test some hypotheses, so he kindly – along with Professor Julie Pasco – allowed me access to some of the data from a very large ongoing study in Victoria. This study, the Geelong Osteoporosis Study (GOS), is now recognised as one of the leading studies in the world focused on both physical and mental health. Led by Professor Pasco, it involves roughly 3000 men and women, from the age of 20 to 90 and even older, who come to our regional hospital for a thorough health assessment every few years. These wonderful people, who give up their time (and their samples!) to help us do research, have contributed so much to our understanding of what factors influence our risk of developing many diseases, and we are so grateful to them. One of the important strengths of this study is that participants are largely representative of the wider Australian population. This means we can relate what we find in this study to the rest of the community.

At the time, back in the early 2000s, there was very little in the way of mental health data in the GOS; most of the information that was collected from participants focused on risk factors for osteoporosis and fractures. There were some data, however, from a small, self-report questionnaire on depressive symptoms, and I used those to test my first hypothesis: that the dietary intake of omega-3 fatty acids and depressive symptoms in women were linked.

Omega-3 fatty acids and mental health

Omega-3 fatty acids are found mainly in seafoods such as oily fish. A number of wonderful scientists, such as Professor Michael Crawford in the United Kingdom and Professor Andrew Sinclair in Australia, had conducted research since the 1970s showing that these were relevant to mental and brain health due to their high abundance in the brain and their importance to brain signalling processes. Another colleague of mine, a US researcher called Captain Joe Hibbeln (he's a legend in the field, known far and wide as Capt'n Joe), had published some very interesting studies in the late 1990s and early 2000s that looked at the average consumption of seafood in various countries and linked it to rates of depression and bipolar disorders.

What Capt'n Joe's studies showed was that countries with a higher consumption of seafood tended to have lower rates of these mental disorders. He also found a link between lower levels of omega-3 fatty acids in breastmilk and postpartum (postnatal) depression. Although other factors might explain these health issues, the associations ('correlations'; see Chapter 5) were very strong and quite consistent, whereas there were no apparent associations with psychotic disorders such as schizophrenia. This suggested that there might be something about these fatty acids that was particularly important to depressive illnesses.

Capt'n Joe's research kickstarted a lot of interest in the potential role of omega-3 fatty acids in depressive disorders and was followed up with some of the first clinical studies to examine whether fish oil supplements could help people with depression. (Now, many years later, the evidence suggests that fish oil supplements are indeed useful for some people with clinical depression and bipolar disorder, but not for everyone.) There were also some intriguing studies from countries such as Finland suggesting that diets low in fish were linked to an increased risk of depression. Seafood is far more commonly consumed in the Nordic countries than in Australia, Britain and the United States, however, so it was unclear whether there would be a link in Australian populations, where the general consumption of fish is pretty low.

My own early studies

To test this idea, I examined the diet and mental health data we had in the GOS from approximately 750 women. This was one of the first studies on this topic and it was a wonderful learning experience (although also challenging, given how impatient I am by nature) to do the slow and detailed work required to – as much as possible – quantify the amount of omega-3 fatty acids in women's diets from seafood and other sources, such as supplements, over a six-year period and link them to their depressive symptoms, taking into account many other factors, such as education, income and other health behaviours, that could affect both fatty acid intake and mental health.

This is something we need to do with any such study, of course. If we find an association between dietary patterns or the intake of certain foods and health, it could be because people who eat a certain way might differ from others with different eating habits because of their income, education, levels of exercise, drinking or smoking habits, or many other such factors. As one example, because fresh fish is sometimes costly, people who eat fish may earn more money than those who don't eat fish. These factors, in turn, are related to the risk of mental disorders such as depression, so we need to take these into account when trying to work out any associations between food and health, including mental health. We use statistics to do this as well. It's lucky I like doing statistics.

So what did we find? We didn't find the link between dietary intake of omega-3 fatty acids and women's depressive symptoms that I'd expected. But we did find a possible reason for this, which was also a concerning fact in its own right: the average intake of these fatty acids was very low and very few women actually consumed anything like the recommended intake of these important oils. This made it challenging for us to detect an association statistically. In fact, we found that more than 95 per cent of the women in our study had less than 0.5 of a gram of these fatty acids per day, which is far less than the roughly 1 gram per day recommended for women. This is pretty similar to data from other Western countries, such as the United States and Britain. Because these fatty acids can't be produced by the body, they need to be consumed in the diet. The fact that so few women were eating enough of these was a real shock to me and made me even more interested in pursuing this line of questioning.

The other reason I was particularly interested in doing further research on this topic – apart from a personal belief that diet is fundamental to every aspect of our health and functioning – was the new evidence from a number of different areas of health research indicating the importance of the immune system to depression, and the emerging field of neuroscience focused on brain plasticity. I'll examine these in more detail in future chapters, but simply speaking, the increasing evidence was that these factors are quite critical to mental health, particularly depression, and that each of these was influenced by diet. For these reasons, I felt sure there would be a link between dietary habits and mental disorders such as depression, and I was determined to find a way to investigate the whole diet and its possible link to mental health.

I set out on a quest to get myself a scholarship so that I could do a PhD to study this question. By this time, I had finished my undergraduate degree in psychology and had commenced an honours year in medical science focusing on epidemiology. This was very challenging because I'd never studied maths, chemistry or biology in senior high school. Oh no, I was going to be an *artist*, so why would I need to study those subjects? (When your child says, 'Why do I need to learn maths – when am I *ever* going to use it?' tell them about me. I regret it every day.)

Anyway, I got myself a medical dictionary and set myself to work to read a (literal) metre-high pile of papers to try to get my head around this medicine business. From sheer stubbornness and hard work (and that wonderful little medical dictionary) I managed to produce a decent thesis and two more papers on depression and both heart and bone health. I was then successful in obtaining a scholarship from the wonderful Australian Rotary Health (thank you, Rotary!) to do my PhD, which I commenced in early 2005. The topic I proposed for my PhD was the possible link between diet and the common mental disorders (depression and anxiety) in Australian women. Although this idea was considered to be rather out there at the time, I had good support from Michael and Julie as my supervisors, and together with another PhD student (hello, Lana) we started on a very ambitious attempt to undertake detailed psychiatric interviews with all the roughly 1000 women in the GOS due to attend the hospital for their ten-year assessments.

In addition to their psychiatric assessments, which examined different manifestations of depression and anxiety disorders, including phobias, post-traumatic stress disorder, generalised anxiety disorder and panic disorder, we also collected detailed data on the women's dietary habits, their physical activity levels, whether or not they smoked, how much alcohol they drank, their educational level and socioeconomic status. We also took into account their body weight.

This was a fascinating process, and I learnt so much about people and what makes them tick. I heard so many life stories, particularly from older women who had lived through wars and tragedies. What I noticed, though, over and over again, was that as women aged, their weight increased and their health declined and they were on more and more medications for cholesterol, blood pressure, pain, arthritis and many other chronic conditions. There would be a few that stood out for their excellent health, though. These were very often older people, some of whom lived on farms or in rural areas, and they all had some things in common. They ate diets high in whole foods (this was a very Anglo-Saxon population, so this meant porridge, tea and 'meat and three veg', essentially), low in junk foods, and stayed physically active (and didn't smoke). It was so striking to me to see – in real life – the long-term outcomes arising from the choices people made about their diets and activity levels.

Roughly four years later, Lana and I finished our slightly more than 1000 interviews, I did all my analyses and I submitted my PhD.

So what did I find?

Diet quality is related to Australian women's mental health

My PhD study showed that women whose diets were generally higher in vegetables, fruit, unprocessed red meats (beef and lamb), fish and whole grains were less likely to have clinically significant depressive or anxiety disorders, whereas those with a more 'Western'-type dietary pattern, higher in processed and unhealthy foods such as meat pies, processed meats, pizza, chips, hamburgers, white bread, sugar and flavoured milk drinks, had more depressive symptoms. These relationships were not explained by any of the other factors we considered and were quite consistent across the age range.

Interestingly, we also identified a third (less common) dietary pattern that was high in fruits and salads plus fish, tofu, beans, nuts, yoghurt and red wine, and this pattern seemed to be weakly associated with *more* depression. This was unexpected and warranted some more investigation, which we undertook. I'll tell you what we found in Chapter 11 (hint: it relates to red meat).

While I, of course, was excited by the findings but not particularly surprised, the rest of the psychiatric community *was* rather surprised. Because this was the first time this link had been examined or shown, the study generated a lot of interest and excitement. Indeed, not only was it published in the leading scientific journal, *The American Journal of Psychiatry*, where it also featured on the front cover, but it was voted number one of the top-ten scientific studies in psychiatry for 2010 by the online resource Medscape. You can imagine how pleased I was about this!

There must have been something in the air; in a lovely bit of serendipity, two other similar studies were published at almost exactly the same time in the other two leading journals in psychiatry research.

Diet quality is related to depression in other populations

The first of these studies, led by another research colleague and (now) friend of mine, Professor Almudena Sánchez-Villegas in

Spain, examined information from more than 10,000 Spanish university graduates participating in a study conducted over many years and focused on the Mediterranean diet.

> ## WHAT IS THE MEDITERRANEAN DIET?
>
> The traditional Mediterranean diet has by far the largest and most consistent evidence base for health benefits. It's high in a wide variety of plant foods, such as colourful vegetables, fruits, a wide variety of leafy greens such as rocket, spinach, dandelion and mustard greens, kale, nettles and purslane (many of which are considered weeds in non-Mediterranean countries, but are wonderfully rich in nutrients and bioactive compounds), wholegrain cereals such as barley, buckwheat, millet, oats, polenta, rice, breads, couscous, and pasta, raw nuts, legumes such as lentils, chickpeas and beans, and lots of olive oil. It also incorporates lots of fish, a little bit of red wine and dairy foods, and a low intake of red meat. Traditionally, of course, this type of diet tended to be home-cooked and eaten with friends and family in a relaxed setting. It's likely that this is one of the many reasons why it's so beneficial.

For this study, the researchers assessed how closely the participants' diets resembled a traditional Mediterranean diet (Spain being, of course, a Mediterranean country). Rather than undertaking a psychiatric assessment, the participants were asked whether they'd been diagnosed with depression by a medical practitioner or were taking antidepressants, which meant the method used to ascertain depression wasn't quite as rigorous as ours. On the other hand, this study had many aspects that made it extremely valuable: first and foremost, it was 'longitudinal' in nature.

This means that diet was assessed at the start of the study and anyone who already reported depression wasn't included in the analysis. Then the people with no previous depression were followed up for more than four years to see who developed depression. This is important, because it's possible that the relationships I saw in my PhD study were due to people eating differently *because* of their mental disorder.

We know that appetite changes are very common in people with depression – some lose their appetites, while others crave sweet and fatty foods. Interestingly, experimental studies in animals show that foods high in fat and sugar actually dampen the stress response; in this way, they may act a bit like a drug or other short-term stress-relieving strategies, such as smoking or drinking too much alcohol. So being able to tease apart cause and effect with a long-term study was very useful.

These researchers found that people whose diets most closely resembled the traditional Mediterranean diet were much less likely to develop depression over the duration of the study. In fact, those participants in the highest categories of the Mediterranean diet score were roughly half as likely to develop depression as those who scored low. This was after considering many other important factors, such as gender, smoking, exercise, marital status, employment status, physical health and any medical conditions. This suggested that eating a Mediterranean-style diet might actually prevent depression occurring in the first place.

Professor Sánchez-Villegas has also found that fatty acids are related to depression. She studied saturated fatty acids, which are mainly found in animal foods such as meat and dairy foods; polyunsaturated fatty acids, found in many plant foods as well as seafood; *trans* fatty acids, artificial fats created as part of the process of making many Western-type foods (cakes, biscuits, pies, margarines); monounsaturated fatty acids, found in avocados, olives, olive oil and nuts; and other culinary oils, such as seed oils, butter and margarine. She found, perhaps unsurprisingly, that both poly- and monounsaturated fats seemed to protect against the development of depression, while the trans fats, which are an established risk factor for heart disease, had a very clear relationship with depression; the more people ate of these types of fats, the more their depression risk increased. This was backed up by another piece of research from the same study, where people who ate foods high in trans fats, such as commercially available muffins, doughnuts and croissants, had an increased risk of developing depression compared to participants who avoided them.

It's reassuring to note that, due to increasing awareness of the danger of processed trans fats to heart health, many countries have reduced or removed them from the food supply. While they were very common – particularly in the American food supply – up until recently, over the last few years they have begun to be phased out and are not now commonly present in most foods in many countries. The exception would be some of the cheaper baked goods (muffins, doughnuts, cakes) found on our supermarket shelves. Watch out for the terms 'vegetable oil' or 'hydrogenated' on the ingredients list, as well as palm oil, the processed form of which is bad for both our health and that of the environment. I once tried a doughnut at an airport from one of those companies that specialises in making them and found that it left my tongue coated with a really unpleasant film of trans fat. Gross.

The third study looking at dietary patterns and depression was conducted by another colleague and friend of mine, Dr Tasnime Akbaraly, in nearly 3500 British public servants. Like the previous study, it followed people over time. The depression risk in people with a more 'wholefoods' dietary pattern, who regularly ate lots of vegetables, fruits and fish, was reduced by roughly a third, while the depression risk in those with higher scores for a Western dietary pattern of sweetened desserts, chocolates, fried foods, processed meats, pies, refined grains and high-fat dairy products was increased by more than 50 per cent. In fact, the results were quite remarkably similar to ours. And again, they did not seem to be explained by other factors, such as income or education, and nor was there evidence that they were the result of people eating differently because of their depressive symptoms.

These three studies had a big impact on the field of psychiatry research, prompting many other researchers around the world to investigate this possible link between overall diet and common mental illnesses.

One of the reasons why the field of what we call Nutritional Psychiatry has advanced so quickly is that there were already many population-based studies that had collected information from people about their diets as well as their mental health, but these two key factors had not previously been put together. Researchers had done a lot of work to examine the role of diet in various physical health conditions, but not in mental health. Because so much information was already collected, it was possible for scientists like me to do the necessary analyses relatively quickly, and this started to result in many papers on the topic. For me personally, having my PhD research published in such a high-profile way meant that I was in a far better position to ask for collaboration with other researchers in Australia and overseas; this allowed me to really fast-track my research program and the development of the evidence base. I passionately wanted to do this, as – to my mind – it was of extreme importance to public health.

Furthering my studies of diet and mental health

While I was doing my PhD, I was lucky enough to spend time in Norway. I had hung around and had a lot of fun in Sweden in my twenties and had a real love for Scandinavia and its modern-day Vikings. I particularly appreciate its wonderful cultures, reflected in their political systems, that puts the health and wellbeing of the population first and foremost and supports equality of the sexes, high-quality child care and parental leave, and access to excellent education and medical care as central rights of all its citizens. The standard of living in these countries is so high and the beauty of the cities and countryside is also exceptional. I had never been to Norway, though, and I was unprepared for how intensely beautiful it is. I spent four months there, working with a fantastic team of researchers, one of whom became one of my PhD supervisors. Because its scientists are well supported by their government funding agencies to do this sort of research for the benefit of the public, Norway, like the rest of Scandinavia, has many rich datasets containing survey information from large numbers of people.

I worked with two wonderful Norwegian researchers, Arnstein Mykletun and Simon Overland, to examine data from the large Hordaland Health Study (HUSK), which had collected information on both diet and mental health from nearly 6000 middle-aged and older adults. On my first visit, during my PhD, I'd only been able to assess whether magnesium intake in the diet was related to mental health, rather than looking at people's overall diet. This is because I was still learning the techniques for measuring whole diet properly. In the meantime, I'd chosen magnesium intake as a marker of healthy diet, because it's found in beans, whole grains, leafy green vegetables and nuts. We know from many studies that people in Western countries don't get enough magnesium in their diets for health, mainly because they don't eat enough of these healthy foods. We, in common with others, found that magnesium intake was related to depression: people who ate less of it had more depressive symptoms.

But of course, it was important to look at diet in its entirety, which I was able to do after completing my PhD. When I revisited Norway and the HUSK data, I found that, in common with our Australian study, people with healthier diets – higher intakes of vegetables, fruit, low-fat dairy, whole grains and fish, and a moderate intake of non-processed red meats – were less likely to suffer from depression, and this was also true for anxiety in women.

Intriguingly, however, we found that the group of men with the healthiest diets were also the ones with more anxiety.

Anxiety and diet: reverse causality?

Why would men with healthy diets have more anxiety? Unfortunately, because the dietary and mental health information was collected at the same time in this study, it's not possible to tease apart cause and effect. However, we think that for some people who are more anxious, this may translate into an increased focus on their health and their diet. There's a fine line between paying attention to your health and your health behaviours (diet and exercise) and becoming obsessively focused on these practices. An eating disorder called orthorexia has become increasingly common in recent years. People afflicted with this disorder become obsessed with eating a healthy diet; they eliminate more and more foods and expand their list of food rules to the extent that it affects their ability to function normally and results in weight loss and – often – malnutrition. People with orthorexia can't break their strict diets without experiencing guilt and distress, and this feeds into a heightened anxiety about food and their own health status. You can see why elevated symptoms of anxiety might co-occur with very healthy eating in some people.

On the other hand, a little bit of anxiety, if it translates into better health behaviours, is not necessarily a bad thing. Another good friend of mine in Canada, Professor Ian Colman, has recently published the results of a large study showing that while depression is associated with an increased risk of early death (this has been shown before – indeed, my Norwegian colleagues showed that depression was roughly equivalent to smoking in increasing the risk for early death), anxiety is associated with reduced risk. One possible reason for this is that people who are more anxious take better care of themselves. Maybe they're more conscientious or have more health anxiety, meaning that they pay attention to their health, visit the doctor, and actually listen to and act on their doctors' advice! Either way, it looks like a bit of anxiety might be a good thing for longevity.

Traditional diets and mental health

Another interesting finding from our Norwegian study was that a traditional Norwegian dietary pattern, with more fish and shellfish, potatoes, fruits, vegetables, milk and yoghurt, bread, pasta, rice, meat, legumes and eggs, was linked to lower rates of depression in men and anxiety in women. This finding – that people consuming diets traditional to their countries and cultures are less likely to have common mental disorders – is also borne out by studies from other countries, such as Japan.

When we think about traditional Japanese diets, we think of healthy foods such as fish, vegetables and seaweed, but within any country there is a range of different dietary habits ranging from good to poor, even if the overall traditional dietary patterns are healthy. This is certainly the case with Japan, which is experiencing a change in dietary habits as multinational food corporations and Western-type snack foods penetrate even this very traditional society where food is revered. In fact, if you visit Japan these days you'll see a big difference in the size and shapes of many younger Japanese people compared to their older counterparts.

My colleagues have repeatedly found that people consuming a healthy Japanese dietary pattern, with higher intakes of traditional vegetables such as cabbage, green leaves, radishes, mushrooms, root vegetables, fish, fruit, green tea, tofu, and fermented foods such as natto (which is unfortunately disgusting if you haven't grown up with it, but very good for you), have fewer depressive symptoms than those who eat a diet lower in these foods. Indeed, in one of the most important studies in this field, published in the *British Journal of Psychiatry* and including information from nearly 90,000 Japanese adults, it was found that those following this type of dietary pattern were half as likely to commit suicide over roughly ten years of follow-up.

Interestingly, however, in these Japanese studies neither the dietary patterns that most looked like a Western diet, being higher in meat, processed meat, bread, dairy products, coffee, black tea and soft drinks, nor the high-seafood dietary patterns, were particularly related to either depression or suicide. The researchers speculated that this might be because Western-style foods are still consumed far less frequently in Japan than elsewhere. They also suggested that once a particular threshold of fish consumption is reached, there is no further benefit to eating more fish. Most countries recommend eating fish two to three times per week, and eating more than this might not have any additional health advantages.

There are now many similar studies from countries as diverse as China, Korea, Iran, France, Greece, Italy and the United States, as well as Australia, Norway and the United Kingdom, all reporting a link between a healthier diet and less depression, and many also showing that unhealthier diets are related to more depression. One of the ways scientists try to answer particular questions is to gather all the studies on a topic (a systematic review) and do a statistical analysis of all the data put together; such studies are called meta-analyses. There have been several of these now (my colleagues and I are getting ready to publish one as I write) and the most recent one confirms that – based on the current evidence from around the world – healthier diets higher in plant foods, fish, and healthy oils from fish and plants, are consistently related to lower levels of depression, while unhealthy diets, higher in manufactured foods with added fats, sugars and salt, are associated with increased depression. A large meta-analysis also confirms that people following a Mediterranean-style diet have roughly a 30 per cent reduction in their risk of developing depression.

The question of weight

Many people assume that the consistent link between diet quality and the risk of developing mental health problems must have something to do with body weight. They assume that if people eat an unhealthy diet, then they get fat and it's being fat that 'causes' the mental health problems. While there are some aspects of truth in that idea, it's doesn't actually appear to be the explanation for the links we see.

First, in all the studies we do, we see that the associations are always independent of body weight. In other words, in our studies linking diet and mental health in the population, when we take body weight into account it doesn't change our findings. That's not to say that unhealthy diets don't lead to overweight and obesity – they do. And nor is it to say that being obese doesn't increase at least the risk of depression – it does (although not necessarily by making people miserable, but rather through obesity's influence on biological systems – more on that later). Depression also increases the risk of obesity – again at least partly through biological processes related to stress hormones. But body weight doesn't explain the links we see between diet quality and mental health. Overweight and obesity are of course important to health outcomes, but they don't seem to be the explanation for the mental health associations we see.

I think there are a few reasons for this. First, the link between diet quality and body weight isn't as clear or consistent as you might imagine. You can probably think of many people you know (or maybe this is even you) who eat a healthy diet – full of whole foods, healthy fats and good quality protein foods – and yet aren't in the ideal weight range. They may even be overweight. In fact, I fell into that category for many years! Similarly, you might know thin people who have a terrible diet, living mainly on junk food and cigarettes, for example. This is also not uncommon. Secondly, I believe that the impact of diet quality on mental and brain health does not work through body weight, but more directly. We'll talk more about the direct effects of unhealthy diet on the brain in the following chapters.

The big message

From all the research to date, we can now safely say that the quality of adults' diets is related to their mental health, and this seems to be the case across a multitude of countries and cultures. In the next chapter we'll turn to the research with young people, in whom mental disorders often first manifest.

Key facts

- Diets higher in whole foods such as vegetables, fruits, wholegrain cereals, beans and legumes, nuts and seeds, fish and olive oil are consistently associated with a reduced risk of depression.
- Diets higher in 'junk' foods, such as sugar-sweetened drinks, fried foods, pastries, doughnuts, packaged snacks, and processed and refined breads and cereals are consistently linked to a higher risk of depression.
- These relationships don't seem to be explained by socio-economic status, education, exercise levels, smoking, alcohol, body weight or other risk factors for heart disease, or by reverse causality.
- We see these relationships in many different countries and cultures, suggesting that there's not just one healthy way to eat.
- Traditional diets, such as traditional Norwegian, Mediterranean or Japanese diets, are all associated with better mental health outcomes.
- Many studies show similar associations between diet quality and anxiety or anxiety disorders, although too much anxiety can result in an obsession with diet that isn't necessarily healthy.

3

Diet and mental health in children and adolescents

When I was 12 I had my first panic attack. I honestly had no idea what it was. I was sitting in class and was suddenly overwhelmed by a strong feeling of dread, as if I'd been told a terrible fact with no way of influencing the outcome. It came completely out of the blue. I don't recall that I was worrying about anything or upset about something in particular. It just happened. This is one of the hallmarks of panic attacks; they come out of the blue when you're not necessarily in a stressful situation. In fact, I used to get them when I was in a deep sleep – waking with a terrible feeling that I was dying. This is not at all uncommon, but it is absolutely horrible. It's particularly terrifying when you don't know what it is. I, like many people who experience panic attacks, thought I had a heart condition. I would have chest pain and pain down my left arm, along with heart palpitations and breathlessness. I experienced these periodically throughout my adolescence, and even when I wasn't having actual attacks I would feel that awful sense of dread very often and my heart would 'flutter' every night.

Looking back, I can remember often struggling to get my breath when I was very young, particularly at night-time when I had to turn off the light and hope that the nightmares didn't come. I didn't have asthma or a chest infection; this was anxiety. By the time I was 14 I had my first episode of major depression. This was even more awful. This sense that all the joy had gone, that there was nothing to look forward to, that the world was a dim, grey and dangerous place. I experienced months at a time like this throughout my adolescence, and it really wasn't fun. Everything, from school to friendships, was a struggle. But my experience is not at all uncommon. Adolescence, particularly around puberty, is one of the main risk periods for the onset of these common mental disorders.

Mental disorders start young

You might remember me saying that half of all mental disorders first manifest in early life, before the age of 14. This information comes from a large study of nearly 10,000 Americans, which also established that three-quarters of mental disorders start by the age of 24. It also found that the average age of onset for anxiety disorders in that study was only six years old. This accords with my experience. To my mind, this fact points to the critical importance of identifying and targeting factors in early life that can be *changed* in order to try to prevent at least some mental disorders before they occur. In this light, I consider the work that we and many others have done regarding a role for diet quality in the mental health of children and adolescents to be particularly important.

It's also very important because it's in young people that we're increasingly seeing the effects of changes to our global diets. As I noted before, 40 per cent of Australian adolescents' calories are coming from ultra-processed foods and at least a quarter of Australians aged four to 18 are already overweight or obese. And also as I noted before, the rates are even higher in some regional areas. The figures are roughly the same in Europe and the United Kingdom. The United States is particularly affected.

Diet is important to mental health in Australian children and adolescents

One of the first things I did once I'd finished my PhD was to undertake a study using data from more than 7000 young Australians, aged ten to 14 and from a wide range of socioeconomic backgrounds around the country, to examine whether this link between diet quality and mental health was also there in young people. To do this, we made two diet-quality scores from the information that had been collected as part of the large Healthy Neighbourhoods Study. Our 'healthy' diet score gave points for having breakfast every day before school, consuming low-fat dairy foods at least once a day, eating two or more serves of fruit per day, and at least four serves of vegetables per day (the data we had were fairly limited). For the unhealthy diet score, we had a bit more information available to us; the score was based on how often the young people ate hamburgers, hot dogs or sausages, potato crisps or savoury snacks, biscuits, doughnuts, cakes, pies or chocolate, sweet drinks such as soft drinks, cordial, flavoured waters and milk, and takeaway foods.

An important aspect of this study was that we could take into account, to a certain extent at least, aspects of young people's behaviour and family environments that may have affected both the way they were eating and their mental health. These included things such as levels of family conflict and disorganised family environments, as well as parental education and income, and young people's level of physical activity, smoking behaviours and attitudes to eating.

What we found was striking: those adolescents in the highest category of 'healthy' diet scores were only half as likely to be depressed as those in the lowest category, while for those in the highest category of 'unhealthy' diet score, the likelihood of depression was increased by nearly 80 per cent compared to those in the lowest category.

Another important finding was that the young people in the higher categories of unhealthy diet were not necessarily the same ones in the lowest categories of healthy diet. This highlights a very important point that we see again and again in our studies: *both low intakes of healthy foods and higher intakes of unhealthy foods appear to be problematic for mental health, and these are usually quite independent of each other.*

Put another way, if a person eats lots of healthy foods but also lots of unhealthy foods, this appears to be – based on our current evidence – problematic for mental health. Similarly, if someone avoided junk and processed foods, but also avoided vegetables, whole grains, fruit, fish and the like, this could also be a problem. This is particularly relevant to young people, who may be getting fed healthy food at home, but then going to the corner shop for sausage rolls, hamburgers, ice creams, chips and similar before or after school. Even worse, they could be getting these foods *at* school! Or consider the child who refuses to eat fruits and vegetables, instead living on a limited diet of 'white foods' (white bread, rice, pasta). They might not necessarily be eating lots of processed and junk foods, but they're certainly not getting the nutrients, fibre and important fats they need to grow a healthy brain. This is not just true for children and adolescents, but for adults as well.

Our finding was backed up by another Australian study, which found that adolescents with a dietary pattern higher in takeaway foods, red meat and sweets had higher levels of what we call 'internalising' and 'externalising' behaviours, which are markers of mental health risk. Internalising behaviours include fearfulness, crying, nightmares and separation anxiety, as well as physical complaints such as stomach aches; while externalising includes anger and aggression, bullying and impulsive behaviours. Because it's not usually possible to get very young people to accurately report their own mental health, we often use parent or teacher reports of these behaviours to try to understand what's going on emotionally for children and young adolescents. It doesn't mean that children displaying these behaviours are all going to go on to suffer mental disorders, but they're useful indicators of vulnerability and emotional distress.

We went on to do another study in young adolescents, again using data that had already been collected from approximately 3000 young Australians by the WHO Collaborating Centre for Obesity Prevention. In this study, we could look forward in time by measuring diet and mental health at one point and then again two years later. The results from this study were also striking: not only did we see that diet quality was associated with adolescent mental health in the same way as in the previous study, but that those young people whose diets improved over the two-year period of the study showed improvements in their mental health, while those whose diets got worse also had worsening psychological health over the same time period.

It's not just true in Australia

Many studies from around the world now indicate that diet quality is related to mental health in young people from different cultures, with different dietary practices. For example, a study in Chinese adolescents showed that higher scores on a 'traditional' dietary pattern, including whole grains, vegetables, fruit, rice and soy products, were related to reduced depression and anxiety, while both an unhealthy 'snacking' dietary pattern and a high-meat dietary pattern were related to more depression and anxiety. In Norway, a high consumption of unhealthy foods was associated with increased behavioural problems in adolescents, while both fruit and fish consumption were associated with fewer behavioural problems. Similarly, a German study reported that an increased intake of sweets was associated with increased emotional symptoms in children compared with a low intake, while a higher diet-quality score was associated with lower levels of emotional symptoms. In Fiji, where the population is rapidly moving away from traditional to Western diets, a study I was involved in showed that young people eating healthier diets, with fruits and vegetables as prominent features, had better mental health. Even after factoring in drug use, smoking, alcohol consumption, social deprivation, family conflict and low social support, another study I led showed that unhealthier diets were linked to more mental health problems in young people from very socially deprived areas of East London.

Our young people need our help

More and more studies are being published pointing to the same thing – diet matters to the mental health of young people. Reflecting this, a recent systematic review bringing all the evidence together concluded that diets higher in unhealthy sugar- and fat-rich foods are related to poor mental health in children and adolescents, while healthier diets are related to better mental health. Given that the majority of mental health problems develop by early adulthood, and that diet is something that affects the entire population and can (definitely) be improved upon, I believe that this new research has clear implications for public health and the prevention of mental disorders. If we think about the nutritional needs of the developing brain, including vitamins, minerals, healthy fats and the like, this shouldn't be at all surprising. But think about the young people in your life – what do they eat? What don't they eat? If you're like the majority of the world's population now, I'm betting their diets are far from optimal. We'll talk about strategies and recommendations for improving things in a later chapter, but in the meantime, it's worth considering where things could be improved for children in your family and community.

Key facts

- There are high levels of both unhealthy diet and mental health problems in young people.
- The quality of adolescents' diets is linked to their mental health, even when we factor in their family environment, social support, drug and alcohol use and other risk factors.
- These associations between both healthy and unhealthy diet and mental health are independent of each other. In other words, unhealthy foods seem to be a risk factor for depression, even if there is also a decent intake of healthy foods. And vice versa.
- Many risk factors for depression in young people are not easily modified, but diet – as well as exercise – is protective for adolescents' mental health and *is* modifiable. This makes it an important target for prevention.

4

Diet at the start of life

Now I'm going to tell you about what I think is possibly the most important research in this new field. Certainly, to my mind, as someone passionately committed to the idea of prevention, these studies are critical to understand and act upon.

Let's go back to the beginning

What happens during pregnancy and in the first few years of life has a substantial influence on physical and mental health outcomes in children. It has been known since the 1980s that poor nutrition, particularly during pregnancy, influences a child's risk of developing chronic disease across their lifespan. Babies born with a low birthweight and/or exposed to malnutrition during in-utero development are at an increased risk of being overweight and of developing heart disease, diabetes, hypertension and stroke in adulthood. This is because what happens in utero 'programs' the developing fetus and influences how the child responds to its environment as it grows.

Food deprivation in early life results in changes to metabolism and an increased tendency to gain weight. In other words, children with stunted growth from having poor nutrition in the womb are at increased risk of becoming overweight or obese as they age. In the past, babies with low birthweight didn't generally go on to gain extra weight as they grew, because access to high-energy foods was limited. As a result, however, of the industrialisation of our food systems even in very poor countries, children now have access to foods that are very high in calories although not necessarily nutritious, and this can result in too much weight gain as they grow. Indeed, a clear link between stunting and overweight/ obesity is seen in children across many countries, including China, Russia, South Africa, South America, Mexico and Brazil, and even in the poorest of African countries.

Stunting from malnutrition during pregnancy has been primarily considered to be due to poverty and a lack of access to food in mothers from developing economies. But there's also some evidence of stunting alongside obesity in children in Western countries, where famine or malnutrition is rare. In a national study conducted in Australia during the early 2000s, nearly 4500 children from a range of socioeconomic backgrounds were assessed. The researchers wanted to see whether children from poorer backgrounds were heavier than their wealthier counterparts, which is a phenomenon seen in many parts of the Western world. As they expected, children from poorer backgrounds had a higher body mass index (BMI) than their peers from middle- and high-income backgrounds. But what was *unexpected* was that these children were also 1–2 centimetres shorter, on average, than wealthier children. This suggests that these Australian children might have experienced stunted growth, just like children in poorer countries. How could this be?

While famine and outright malnutrition are rare in most Western countries nowadays, and certainly in Australia, what's not rare is what's known as malnubesity. This refers to a situation where too much energy is consumed but that energy comes with very little nutrition. The ultra-processed foods that make up so much of the modern diet are high in calories from fats and sugars but very low in nutrients, which means they make people fat without actually providing the nutrition needed for all the body's processes, including growth. And so the current food environment has given rise to a common situation where individuals are both overweight or obese *and* undernourished. And this suggests that may not be only low birthweight and outright lack of food during gestation that's an issue for children's later health and growth, but the consumption of our modern Western diets during pregnancy. And this may be relevant not only to obesity and chronic diseases, but to mental disorders as well.

Very important studies by Professor Ezra Susser and colleagues at Columbia University in the United States have shown that people conceived during the height of the Dutch Hunger Winter in 1944–45, when daily rations allowed for less than 900 calories per day and more than 20,000 people died of famine-related causes, had an increased risk of schizophrenia, as well as depressive and bipolar disorders. This strongly suggests that malnutrition has a profoundly negative impact on brain development, which is probably not surprising. As I said, malnutrition from lack of food is rare in Western countries; however, given the commonness of 'malnubesity', it made sense to me that unhealthy diets in early life might be related not just to children's physical health, but also their mental health.

Diet during pregnancy is related to children's emotional health

In 2011, I successfully applied for an award from a large US philanthropic organisation, NARSAD, to test the idea that early-life nutrition is related to children's emotional health. This allowed me to return to Norway, this time to investigate data from a *very* large study of mothers and their children – the Norwegian Mother and Baby Cohort Study (known as MoBa). I worked with my colleagues there to examine information on the diets of more than 23,000 women during their pregnancy, and also on their children's diet in the first years of life. We wanted to see if there was a link between mothers' diets during pregnancy, children's diets, and children's emotional health, measured by assessing internalising and externalising behaviours from the ages of 18 months to five years. Questionnaires completed by parents and other caregivers about these behaviours can give us information about the emotional health of even very young children.

It was a wonderful experience to go back to Norway – this time to Oslo – to join my colleagues on this study. You can just imagine the effort involved in getting so many data together and analysed, but I was lucky enough to work with an amazing statistician who was able to wrestle all the information into a form we could use to test our hypothesis and present our results in a useful way. We needed to take into account all the sorts of things that might affect a mother or child's diet, as well as the children's mental health. These were factors such as how old the mother was, how many other children she had, her parenting style, the educational level and income of the family, whether the mother was partnered or alone, and – very importantly – the mother's mental health during pregnancy. What we wanted to see was the trajectory over time of these internalising and externalising behaviours in young children, related back to the mothers' diets during pregnancy, but also to their own diets in those special first few years.

We worked hard and generated some fascinating results, which were for the most part in line with what I had expected. We found that children whose mothers had an unhealthier dietary pattern during pregnancy, with more processed meat products, refined cereals, sweet drinks and salty snacks, had higher levels of externalising behaviours, quite independently of what the children themselves ate over those first few years of life. But the quality of the children's diets was also related to their emotional health: children who ate fewer healthy foods, such as white and oily fish, vegetables, fruit, eggs and Norwegian bread (which is lovely dark whole grain), and/or more foods such as chips, buns, cakes, waffles, chocolate, cookies, sweets, soda, diet soda, ice cream and pizza, had more emotional health problems, reflected in higher levels of both internalising and externalising behaviours. These relationships between children's diets and their emotional health existed quite independently of the quality of their mothers' diets. In other words, what mothers ate *and* what children ate were both related to children's emotional health. And these relationships were independent of all those other things I mentioned, the most important of which was likely to be the mothers' depression and anxiety symptoms.

We know that the children of mothers with depression are more at risk of having mental health problems themselves, whether through genetics, exposure to stress hormones during gestation, or the impact of the mothers' behaviour and parenting practices. This is an important point that we'll come back to shortly. We did find a clear link between the mothers' mental health and that of their children, but we were also surprised to find a similarly clear link between the children's diet and their emotional health. This suggests that diet during pregnancy and early life might be an important factor in a child's risk of later mental problems. And of course, diet is something we can control and improve.

As I mentioned, our results were pretty much in line with what I'd hypothesised, with one important exception. The children of mothers with particularly healthy diets during their pregnancies had *more* internalising behaviours. Why might this be? We discussed earlier that there's a link between anxiety and health behaviours and that internalising behaviours in children reflect worry and anxiety. We think our results might be evidence that anxious mothers produce anxious children (which we already knew) and that the mothers' dietary habits were – at least partly – a result of their tendency to be anxious. So although in our study eating a healthy diet during pregnancy didn't seem to be necessarily protective of children's mental health, eating an unhealthy diet during pregnancy *did* seem to be problematic. And the children eating an unhealthy diet during the first few years of life was definitely an issue.

In the following year, two more studies examined this link between what mothers eat during pregnancy and children's emotional health. In the Netherlands, a large study called Generation R examined mothers' diets and children's mental health in approximately 3000 Dutch mother–child pairs. In contrast to what we found, this study showed that a diet higher in vegetables, fruits and fish during pregnancy was associated with better emotional health in children over the first few years of life. In other words, a healthy diet during pregnancy seemed to be protective. They also showed that the children of mothers who ate a 'traditional Dutch' diet during pregnancy, higher in fresh and processed meats, potatoes and margarines, had more emotional problems.

Finally, another important study from King's College in London also backs up our findings: using information from the large Avon Longitudinal Study of Parents and Children (ALSPAC) in the United Kingdom, researchers examined levels of depressive symptoms in nearly 8000 pregnant women to see whether this was related to the healthiness or otherwise of their own diets and that of their children's diets in the early years. The researchers wanted to understand whether poor mental health during pregnancy might have had an impact on the way mothers ate and what they fed their children once they were born. They also wanted to investigate whether the mothers' or the children's diets were subsequently related to the children's emotional health, in a similar way to our study. Because ALSPAC is also a very high-quality study, the researchers were again able to consider many very important factors that might have affected both the mothers' diets and their and the children's emotional health, including poverty, adequacy of housing and living conditions, being the sole caregiver, the mothers' educational level, and whether or not the mother had been involved with the police or subject to domestic violence.

Unsurprisingly perhaps, these researchers found that mothers who had more depression also had unhealthier diets during pregnancy and fed their children less healthy diets during the first years of life. This has been observed before, particularly in mothers from disadvantaged backgrounds. Children of the mothers with more depressive symptoms also had more emotional problems, also as expected. But in common with the previous studies, they also found that eating an unhealthy diet during pregnancy was directly related to more emotional problems in children over the first seven years of life, and this wasn't explained by the mothers' mental health or other potentially important factors.

How does early life affect children's emotional health?

While I'm going to discuss the mechanisms linking diet and mental and brain health in more detail later on, it's worth having a quick look here at the different ways diet in early life could affect emotional health in children. While nutrient deficiencies during pregnancy can affect brain development, other aspects of food and diet during pregnancy appear to have an impact on the developing brain. To understand this better, we need to look at studies in animals where researchers are able to carefully manipulate and control diet and examine the impact on brain and behaviour in close detail.

In such studies, sugary and/or high-fat diets fed to pregnant animals, such as mice or non-human primates (e.g. chimpanzees), reduce brain plasticity (the growth of new nerve cells) in the region of the brain called the hippocampus, which we know is central to learning and memory and also important in mental health. Such diets also affect the neurotransmitter systems in offspring, reducing levels of serotonin, popularly known as a 'happy hormone', and increasing anxiety-like and aggressive behaviours, even when the animals become adults. Deficiencies in those very important omega-3 fatty acids (from fish and seafood) also reduce the plasticity of the brain and increase anxiety behaviours in the next generation.

Unhealthy diets during pregnancy also affect the reward systems in developing brains. Researchers believe that this influences the transmission of obesity through generations: eating junk food during pregnancy seems to make the children more responsive to the pleasure they get from eating such foods. In addition, junk-food-style diets during pregnancy not only activate the stress-response system, which can make animal offspring more hyperactive, but also change immune-system functioning. Given the immune system of the body and brain is closely linked to the expression of mental disorders such as depression, this is likely to be important. High-fat diets in mothers can also shape the gut microbiota of the offspring (see Chapter 8 for more). Finally, such diets given to animals during pregnancy have a detrimental effect on the parenting behaviours of those animals once their babies are born, and this also makes sense in light of the evidence we now have concerning diet during pregnancy and the *mothers'* mental health.

Several studies have shown that mothers who eat more healthily during their pregnancy are less likely to experience postnatal depression. For example, in the ALSPAC study, mothers whose diets were lower in healthy foods and/or higher in unhealthy foods during pregnancy had higher depressive symptoms in the postnatal period. Similarly, a study in Greece showed that mothers consuming a healthier (Mediterranean-style) diet during pregnancy were only half as likely to have postnatal depression as those with the lowest diet scores. Because mothers' mental health is closely linked to their children's mental health, this is also another important reason to focus on mothers' diets during pregnancy. We'll discuss this concept further and in more detail in later chapters.

My own pregnancy story

When I was pregnant with my first daughter, my diet was appalling in the first three months or so. Even though I normally ate a pretty healthy diet, I was *so* sick with morning sickness that I felt like I had a scale-ten hangover 24 hours a day. It was really hideous. And like many people with a hangover, all I wanted to eat was chips and ice cream. It was pretty terrible (and I put on a lot of weight). Of course, this was way before I'd done my research and there wasn't any information out there to suggest that this might be a problem for my baby. As it happens, Phoebe suffered from quite bad anxiety and depression during her adolescence, although she's emerging from that now as she becomes an adult. Was it my fault? Who knows? I had a strong personal and family history of depression, so she might just have inherited that tendency. It might also be that because I'm an anxious person, I was worried almost every minute of the day during my pregnancy with her. Being exposed to lots of stress hormones during gestation is *not* good for babies, so maybe that was the reason. We'll never know whether my diet had anything to do with it or not, but it does highlight a very important point.

Don't blame yourself

Many people, when I tell them about the research evidence linking diet during pregnancy to mental (and physical) health outcomes in children, suggest that I'm just providing another reason for mothers to feel guilty. As if we don't have enough of these already! My response, however, is that we shouldn't be blaming ourselves, but rather the food environment, which makes eating unhealthy foods so much easier and cheaper than eating whole foods. This is where we need to be focusing our blame – not on mothers. More about that later.

The links between diet and mental health are clear

If we bring all the research from the past few years together, it's clear that habitual diet quality is related to the risk of developing common mental and emotional health problems, particularly depression, in children, adolescents and adults. These associations don't seem to be explained by other factors such as income, marital status, where people live, education, body weight, other cardiometabolic risk factors, how much people exercise or drink alcohol, or whether or not they smoke. The links aren't explained by people's mental health prompting changes in their diets either, as far as we can tell.

The fact that this association is apparent in people from countries as diverse as Japan, Norway, Australia, China, Spain, France, Brazil, the United States and the United Kingdom highlights an important point: a healthy Japanese or Chinese diet might differ in its details from a healthy Norwegian or Spanish diet, but they all have at their core a higher intake of plant foods and 'whole' foods – that is, foods that haven't been processed, packaged, added to, subtracted from or otherwise interfered with.

Many people get hung up on the details of diet, worrying that if they do or don't include particular foods their health will suffer. The truth is that we don't have sufficient evidence to say one sort of healthy diet is superior to another for any particular person, although I do think we're getting closer to being able to do that. As long as our daily diet includes a diversity of plant and other unprocessed foods, we'll be way ahead of the pack in our health. Of course, it's critical to avoid as much as possible the foods at the other end of the spectrum, and we know what they are. Needless to say, I'm a big fan of journalist and author Michael Pollan's recommendation, with one small clarification: *'Eat [whole] foods, not too much, mostly plants.'* Keep it simple!

Key facts

- Early-life nutrition is linked to both physical and mental health outcomes in children.

- The quality of mothers' diets during pregnancy is related to their children's emotional health, independent of a wide range of potentially explanatory factors.
- Children's diets during the early years are also related to their emotional health, independent of their mothers' diets and other family factors, such as education, family environment and income.
- The impact of an unhealthy diet on children's emotional health may result from changes in many bodily systems, such as the hippocampus, the immune system, neurotransmitter systems, the stress-response system and the gut.
- Mothers' diets are related to mothers' mental health, which is also very important to children's mental health.

5

Correlation doesn't equal causation: a brief but important note about science

There are many challenges to conducting dietary research, and I want to mention just a few of them so that you're in a better position to evaluate the evidence and make your own decisions about nutrition and health.

First and foremost, most of the studies in this field of Nutritional Psychiatry so far are based on what we call epidemiological or 'observational' studies. These, simply speaking, involve collecting information from large groups of people who (we hope) are representative of their populations or communities, and then using statistics to test hypotheses about which risk factor is related to which health outcome. In these studies, as I mentioned, we do our best to account for the many different factors that might influence both diet and mental health, but the reality is that it's not always possible to capture with questionnaires the subtleties and nuances of these factors (such as social disadvantage, family environments, parenting practices and other health behaviours). It's also possible that we're missing information on some crucial third factor or factors that might explain the links that we see. For example, there might be genetic factors that predispose people to both eating badly and having poor mental health!

It's also the case that many of the studies in this new field have been 'cross-sectional', meaning that we collect the dietary data and the mental health data at the same time. This means that we can't then exclude the possibility that the dietary habits we see are a *result* of mental health rather than a cause. This is called 'reverse causality'. Although many other studies in this area *have* been prospective, meaning that we collect the dietary information at the start and then 'follow' people to see who develops mental health problems, it's not always possible to fully tease apart cause and effect when it comes to health and health behaviours.

The other big problem is the measurement of diet, which is very prone to misreporting and, thus, what we call 'measurement error'. Almost everyone is pretty appalling at accurately remembering or recording their food intake for research studies, particularly when it comes to estimating their overall energy intake. In fact, the more overweight people are, the more likely they are to under-report calorie or unhealthy food intake (although I suspect it's not deliberate, but rather wishful thinking). Such measurement error can make it very difficult to get an idea of what foods and dietary patterns are related to health, and how important diet might be. When we see discrepancies in the data, it's quite likely caused – at least in part – by measurement error. There is a *lot* of effort going into new phone apps and computer programs that can capture the information from photographs of meals to give a more accurate insight into what people actually eat, but in the meantime we're stuck with pretty inexact ways of measuring diet. Happily, these do still seem to be useful for ranking people on how healthy or unhealthy their diets are.

On the other hand, there are so many studies in this field now and, with a very few exceptions, they point to the same thing: diet is an important component in the risk of developing common mental health problems throughout life. Indeed, I'm somewhat amazed at how consistent the findings are, given the methodological challenges. Many of the longitudinal studies, where people have been followed up over time, have also investigated the reverse-causality hypothesis in some detail and have found that this doesn't explain the associations they see. In fact, we analysed data from a longitudinal study of adults in Australia and found that – contrary to our expectations – people who had previously experienced depression (but didn't have depression at the time of the first assessment) actually had *healthier* diets than those who had never had depression! We know from another Australian survey that many people make efforts to improve their diets in an attempt to treat their own depressive symptoms. This points to the reality, I think, that people intuitively know that what they feed themselves translates to how they feel.

Having said all of that, the only way we can really get at 'causality' is to do experiments. There have been many, many experiments using animals, and they tell us that dietary components, including high-fat and/or high-sugar diets, berries and other foods high in antioxidants, and omega-3 fatty acids, have an impact on the brain – particularly in promoting or reducing 'neuroinflammation' and brain plasticity. We need to do experimental studies in people, however, to know whether the findings from these animal studies translate to humans.

Such studies are particularly challenging in humans for a number of reasons. First and foremost, we can't blind people to the nature of the experiment. If we're testing a medication, the gold-standard approach is a double-blind, randomised, placebo-controlled trial, where neither the person receiving the medication, nor the study personnel (including the assessors and the statistician) know whether the participant was taking the medication or the placebo until after the study has closed and the data have been analysed. This is important because we know that the placebo response is very powerful, and that if people believe they're getting a treatment that's going to help them, it often does help, whether or not it has any therapeutic effect! It's also worth noting that there's something called the 'nocebo' response, when a person believes that whatever they're taking – be it a drug or other treatment, or a food containing gluten or MSG, for example – is going to have a negative impact on their health or symptoms and they similarly manifest these. The brain is an amazing thing and the placebo/nocebo response is a particularly interesting aspect of medicine.

Needless to say, however, this presents particular problems for nutritional experiments in psychiatry (or any other nutritional health research), where it's very difficult to blind people to the nature of the diet they're eating, and where the participants' expectations of benefit could influence their mental health symptoms. It's also unethical, of course, to put some people on a junk-food diet for any length of time to see what happens! And it would be very problematic to lock people up for a number of weeks and feed them only what we wanted to feed them. To get at the true influence of diet on mental health we would ideally need to put a large number of people out in the community on a very tightly controlled diet for a reasonable length of time and follow them closely. This presents all sorts of expense and logistical challenges, not least in getting people to adhere to a diet over the long term (it's hard enough for even the most committed of us).

For these reasons, the field of Nutritional Psychiatry has only just started to conduct experimental studies; we will cover these in Chapter 9.

Finally, there's something that is very important to understand about the recommendations you might get from medical doctors, other health professionals, or friends and family, which are very often based on clinical or personal experience rather than on good-quality research studies conducted with the necessary rigorous scientific methodologies. This relates to the placebo response, but also 'confirmation bias' and something called 'regression to the mean'.

Confirmation bias is fairly simple to understand – unconsciously, we tend to pay more attention to, or believe, information or advice that conforms to our prior expectations or beliefs. For example, if we read that a particular food is associated with a particular health benefit, and that's in line with what we already believed, then we're more likely to remember that advice and act on it. If, on the other hand, we read that that food is actually associated with a negative effect and this is contrary to our beliefs, we're less likely to have faith in it or to remember or act upon it. This is just human nature.

This is also true for our experiences when we're ill, and this is where 'regression to the mean' is important to understand. What does this term mean? Most acute illnesses follow a course, where they have a lead-up period as we develop the illness, the zenith of the illness when we're really feeling our worst, then the recovery phase. Even chronic illnesses tend to wax and wane with a similar trajectory. Of course, when we're really feeling our worst is when we tend to go to the doctor or our chosen health professional. We don't generally go to see them when we're getting worse ('Maybe I'll feel better tomorrow, or next week,' we tell ourselves, 'so I'll just hold off for a while . . .') and we don't go to see them when we're getting better; we usually go to see them (or visit the chemist or health food shop) when we're at our sickest.

So when we're told to take (or we self-prescribe) a certain food or supplement X, Y or Z, and then we recover from what ails us in line with the normal illness trajectory, we will of course attribute our recovery to whatever action or substance it was that we took. This is also true for clinicians – even medical doctors, who are often not trained in research and so are less well placed to evaluate findings from research studies. They'll attribute their patients' recovery to the prescription or advice they gave – which is also human nature. Or they'll base their recommendations on the similar clinical experiences of their colleagues.

The trouble is that this isn't evidence that something does or doesn't work. A multitude of background factors that are changing all the time could explain why someone does (or doesn't) recover from an illness – one of the main ones is that they would be recovering anyway (regression to the mean). But they might also have had a few nights of better sleep, or a stressful life event might have resolved, or an unrecognised virus or bacterial infection that had been ticking on in the background might have abated, or one of the other medications or supplements they might be taking or dietary changes they might have made, or any one of a million other small things that happen in our complex lives, might have been the cause of the change in illness status.

The only real way to know if something affects a health outcome is by conducting high-quality double-blind, placebo-controlled trials. And where these are not feasible (no one has ever run a double-blind, placebo-controlled trial, for example, to confirm that smoking causes cancer, for very obvious reasons) then we have to rely on multiple avenues of evidence from many different types of studies, including animal experiments, observational studies, and real-world 'pragmatic' trials. This is what I and my colleagues are now attempting at Deakin University's Food & Mood Centre, but the field is young and we need far more research to really 'know' the answers to a lot of our questions. It's important to keep these caveats in mind when reading about the studies in this new field, as well as in the wider field of medical and nutrition research.

And please keep this in mind when you read pronouncements from the self-proclaimed diet 'experts' and bloggers. Just because everyone eats doesn't mean that everyone is an expert on diet. It's very important that we rely on research evidence for our guidelines and recommendations, not on those who think they know because of a few scientifically iffy studies, their personal experience, or that of their patients.

6

Autism, ADHD and psychotic illnesses

In the previous chapter, we discussed the evidence for a link between nutrition throughout life and the risk of developing what we call the common mental disorders – depression and anxiety. We also talked about the relationship between the quality of a child's nutrition during early life, including during their in-utero development, and their risk of developing emotional health problems in childhood. But does early-life nutrition, apart from outright malnutrition as in the Dutch Hunger Winter studies, have a bearing on other mental disorders such as autism spectrum disorder (ASD), attention deficit hyperactivity disorder (ADHD), or psychotic disorders such as schizophrenia?

This is an important question, but a difficult one to answer for two reasons. First, these disorders have a big neurodevelopmental component. This means that they arise, at least in part, from problems that occurred as a child's brain was developing, most likely in combination with events or exposures in early life and also, of course, their genetic make-up. There's even evidence now that the parents' health (yes, dad's as well) *before* pregnancy might play a role in these disorders. So our studies need to pay very close attention to the parents' health and what they're doing both before and during pregnancy, as well as the child's early-life family environment. This is challenging.

Secondly, because these disorders are rarer than the common mental disorders or emotional problems in young people, we need far larger studies carried out over a very long period of time to work out any dietary connections. We would need to start with a very large group of parents during (or even before) pregnancy, gather very good-quality information from them, and follow their children over a long period to see which of the children develops these sorts of disorders. Then track back to examine the information on what the parents ate before and during their pregnancy, taking into consideration all sorts of other factors that can affect both nutrition and mental and brain health.

Luckily, versions of such studies do exist – the MoBa and ALSPAC studies are two good examples. Although the children from these studies are generally not yet old enough to have developed psychotic disorders, which tend to manifest in late adolescence and early adulthood, they are old enough to yield information on their cognitive (brain) and emotional health. From these studies, we're starting to get an inkling of which nutritional factors might play a role.

Diet quality during pregnancy is linked to brain health in children

We've already discussed the link between mothers' diets during pregnancy and their children's emotional behaviour. In a similar vein, a very recent meta-analysis by our Norwegian colleagues has assessed all the evidence in this new field and concluded that the children of mothers who have better quality diets during pregnancy *are* more likely to have better emotional health. They also found that better diets during pregnancy, with higher intakes of vegetables, fruits and particularly fish, produce children with better cognitive health – in other words, their general intelligence (IQ), language, motor skills development, problem-solving and personal–social skills. Finally, they found that better diets during pregnancy are related to reduced symptoms of ADHD, ASD and conduct disorders in children.

We're currently using the very large MoBa study to examine maternal diets and ADHD and ASD in more detail. This should give us more insights, but the evidence at this stage all indicates that the better the nutrition during pregnancy, the better the brain health of the developing child. It's worth noting that the majority of studies that have examined this question have focused on the consumption of fish during pregnancy. This is due to the recognised importance of the omega-3 fatty acids to the brain and brain development. But people who eat more fish also tend to eat more healthy foods on average, so the researchers also used fish intake as a marker of a healthy diet.

These findings shouldn't be surprising, given the importance of good nutrition to healthy development in general, but it's not entirely clear which is more important – the mother's diet or the child's. Only a few studies have examined this particular question, although more are underway. This relative lack of information partly relates to the difficulty of measuring diets, given how poor people are at accurately recording what they or their children eat.

These studies are all 'observational' in nature, which means we can't conclusively say that diet has a *direct* effect on child emotional and/or brain health. It's not particularly feasible to conduct experiments on large groups of pregnant women to see whether a particular diet has an effect on children's health and wellbeing as they age. (Can you imagine getting ethical board approval to put pregnant women on a junk-food diet? Or the difficulties involved in getting large numbers of women to adhere rigorously to a particular diet for their whole pregnancy?) So, until we can figure out how to do the science, we're limited to these sorts of observational studies.

But there is another, potentially more accurate way of examining diet, and that is to study the metabolic health of parents before and during pregnancy.

Metabolic health in parents is related to children's health

Throughout her pregnancy, a woman is usually in the care of medical practitioners – obstetricians, nurses and the like. Her physical health is monitored, and in many countries her blood glucose, blood pressure and other aspects of her physical health will be measured. She will also be weighed regularly both to make sure the baby is growing and to see whether she is gaining enough weight (or too much weight) over the course of her pregnancy. These sorts of clinical measurements are much more accurate than asking people about their regular diets. What is useful for us to know is that whether or not a mother has gestational diabetes or high blood glucose, hypertension (high blood pressure), or puts on too much body weight in pregnancy is – to some extent at least – related to the quality of her diet both before and during pregnancy. Although this is a less direct way of looking at diet, it's helpful to consider what we know about metabolic health in parents and its relationship to children's health outcomes, particularly as there's quite a bit of research in this area.

While we've already discussed the evidence that babies with low birthweight are at increased risk of heart disease, type 2 diabetes and obesity as they age, particularly if they're exposed to an obesogenic environment in childhood, it's also the case that large-for-gestational age (LGA) infants are at increased risk of childhood obesity, which can lead to insulin resistance, type 2 diabetes and hypertension later in life. Obese mothers are more likely to give birth to LGA infants, *particularly* if they are obese when they first become pregnant. In other words, the mother's weight before pregnancy might be even more important than any weight gain during pregnancy in influencing the child's weight at birth. Of course, a mother's weight before pregnancy is also an indicator of her long-term dietary habits.

Women who are obese when their child is conceived are more likely to have children with congenital abnormalities, such as neural tube defects, as well as a number of other problems related to development, including oral clefts, heart anomalies and hydrocephaly (fluid on the brain). We don't completely understand why or how obesity before and during pregnancy might lead to congenital abnormalities, but it's thought to relate to poor glucose metabolism – which is strongly influenced by diet. One large study found, for example, that mothers who ate a diet higher in sugar and high-glycemic-index foods (refined carbohydrates) were twice as likely to have children with neural tube defects, and four times as likely if the mothers were also obese. Why is this so important? Because at least a third of pregnant women in the United States are obese, and obesity before and during pregnancy is becoming increasingly common across the globe.

I have a close friend who is a midwife in a small-town hospital in the United States. She tells me that morbid obesity in the mothers is now so common that they have had to design a contraption *to hold women's stomachs up and out of the way* so that the surgeons can do the caesareans that are so often necessary when mothers are obese. Just think about that for a minute.

Western diets also cause type 2 diabetes, which is becoming increasingly common across the world. New research shows that the growth of the heads, limbs and abdomens of fetuses in diabetic mothers differs from those fetuses from non-diabetic mothers, which again indicates the importance of blood glucose regulation in mothers. In addition, putting (non-diabetic) pregnant women on low-glycemic-load diets, made up of unprocessed wholegrains, vegetables, fruits, beans, nuts and yoghurt, has been shown to reduce their glycemic response to meals and to improve their insulin sensitivity, while a diet consisting of carbohydrates from refined breads and breakfast cereals, desserts and snack foods made things worse, particularly in the later stages of pregnancy, when mothers' blood glucose levels have the greatest impact on fetal growth.

The evidence tells us that mothers' metabolic health, and likely their diets, are linked to the risk of physical abnormalities in infants, but what about brain health? An important US study investigated diabetes (type 2 or gestational), obesity, and high blood pressure in pregnant women and found that these metabolic conditions were more common in the mothers of children with ASD and developmental delay; indeed, mothers with diabetes were more than twice as likely to have a child with developmental delays, and mothers with a metabolic disorder (not necessarily diabetes) were more likely to have children with impairments in visual reception, motor skills, and receptive and expressive language, as well as adaptive communication and socialisation skills.

Another large study that involved more than 12,000 children from Sweden, Finland and Denmark found that children of mothers who were overweight or obese before pregnancy, or who were overweight to start with and then gained too much weight during their pregnancy, were more likely to have symptoms of ADHD than their peers with healthy-weight mothers. Another Swedish study also showed that pre-pregnancy overweight or obesity was linked to more attention problems and emotional behaviours in five-year-olds, while a Finnish study showed that 11-year-old children whose mothers were obese immediately before pregnancy were nearly three times more likely to have an intellectual disability. This again suggests that it's not just what happens in pregnancy, but *before* pregnancy that might be important. And guess what? It's not just the mums we need to be concerned about.

It's not only mums . . .

Another very important piece of research from the large Norwegian MoBa study, including data from more than 90,000 parents and their offspring, showed that the children of obese fathers were at increased risk of developing autism and Asperger's syndrome. In fact, there was a linear relationship, so that the higher the fathers' BMI, the greater the risk. Intriguingly, although mothers' obesity was also related to an increased risk of these disorders, the fathers' weight seemed to be more strongly related to the children's outcomes than the mothers' weight. We had always assumed that only mothers' health and what happens in utero were relevant to children's neurodevelopment, but this study suggests that we need to be looking more widely to understand the mechanisms linking parental lifestyle and body weight to the children's risk of developing these disorders.

One possibility is that the link is due to genetics, as there are genes that increase the risk of both ASD and morbid obesity and these might be transmitted by the fathers. Another possible explanation relates to what we call epigenetics, a field of research that's generating a lot of interest and new evidence. We'll go into this in more detail in Chapter 8, but simply speaking, epigenetics examines the ability of environmental factors, such as diet, to influence gene activity.

Epigenetic changes can be transmitted to the offspring, including via the fathers' sperm. One intriguing experiment in animals showed that feeding a low-folate diet to male rodents before conception resulted in multiple changes in the sperm epigenome (molecules associated with DNA that can influence gene activity), and that the offspring showed changes in genes involved in the development of the central nervous system and in chronic diseases, including diabetes and cancer. This suggests that the diet of the father may affect the information that is transmitted to the fetus, thus influencing the child's development and long-term disease risk.

An important caveat

Most of the existing human studies are based on observational evidence, which means we can't be sure that the metabolic status of parents is *causing* neurodevelopmental and other health problems in children. Although researchers do their best to account for these, it's always possible that other unmeasured or incompletely measured factors increase the risk of both metabolic disorders in parents and poor health outcomes in children. The available evidence does, however, indicate pretty strongly that parental overweight, obesity and high blood glucose are problematic for child health outcomes. And so there is good reason to focus our efforts on giving young people the best chance to be healthy before they become parents themselves, in order to avoid the intergenerational transmission of disease.

A recent series in the leading medical journal, *The Lancet*, focused on exactly this issue. The authors noted that more than 95 per cent of young women in the United Kingdom have dietary intakes of folate and iron that are below the recommendations for healthy pregnancies. Some of the researchers stated:

> Research is now showing that our gametes and early embryos are sensitive to a variety of environmental conditions including poor parental diet. These effects can change the process of development, affecting growth, metabolism and health of offspring, so makes the case for both parents to have a healthy lifestyle well before conception and pregnancy.

and

> We have a large amount of evidence that shows the preconception period is of paramount importance in helping the next generation be healthier in ways that drive down rates of obesity, diabetes and other non-communicable diseases. The good news is that this involves everyone. We need an approach that involves all aspects of society – government, schools, medical professionals, aspiring parents and today's teenagers. It is everyone's responsibility to support our young adults to become successful parents of healthy, long-lived children.

The adolescent brain

Adolescence is a time when a young person undergoes substantial physical changes. There is a surge in the growth of new neurons (nerve cells) in the brain before puberty, which are then 'rewired and pruned' throughout puberty, adolescence, and early adulthood. This results in increased cognitive flexibility, reasoning and planning ability, and improved impulse control, all of which makes the young person better able to respond to their environment. But it also means that the adolescent brain during this time is particularly vulnerable to damaging exposures that can disturb brain development. Of course, adolescence is also a time of increasing independence, when young people begin to make their own food choices and have their own spending money. And we know that the choices they're making are very poor.

As we've seen, in Australia, roughly 40 per cent of the calories young people consume come from highly processed junk foods. These foods interact with the reward systems in the brain, which are particularly receptive at this age. In fact, there's much higher signalling in the reward systems of the brain of adolescents compared with adults, and this is linked to more reward-seeking behaviours. These systems are the same as those that drugs, alcohol and cigarettes act upon. Tasty junk foods – deliberately manufactured with lots of the sugars and fats that we've evolved to crave – give adolescents pleasurable feedback that makes these foods very hard to resist.

Young people are also less able to control their behaviour (to say no to these foods), because the parts of their brains that are used for impulse control are less mature. In animal studies, high-fat and high-sugar foods change the signalling of the dopamine (reward) system, which prompt changes in other neurotransmitters that are critical to higher order thinking. These foods also appear to impair social interactions and behavioural control. In a recent intervention study in human adolescents, boys who were fed large volumes of sugar-sweetened fizzy drinks had poorer impulse control on behavioural tests. This impact of diets high in fat and sugar on impulse control is also supported by evidence from animal research.

Of course, there are strong social norms at this age that also feed into poor eating habits; young people don't have the money to congregate at cafes selling healthy foods, and these are not usually set up to encourage teenagers to 'hang out', but teenagers *do* use fast-food chains as a meeting place. (Indeed, the fast-food outlets bank on it!) What are the implications of this for their developing brain?

First, these foods do, of course, lead to weight gain in many people. But we also need to consider another important point: because children and adolescents are growing rapidly, they're typically 'hungrier', but they're also less likely to put on weight from eating the wrong sorts of foods because they have a faster metabolism and are often (but certainly not always) more physically active. This means that they, and their parents, might not recognise that damage is being done *even if they're not putting on excess weight*. Indeed, there's now experimental evidence that the negative impacts on brain function from junk food can occur before weight gain is apparent.

While we've known for a while that alcohol and cannabis have a negative effect on young people's developing brains and cognitive abilities, we now believe that this may also be true for junk food. From many experiments in animals, we know that performance on memory tasks (the ability to learn new facts) appears to be quickly disrupted by high-fat and high-sugar diets. These foods interact with both the prefrontal cortex and the hippocampus; the hippocampus is the seat of learning and memory in the brain and is important for mental health as well. We also know that these sorts of foods can impact the hippocampus and cognitive abilities independently of body weight, and the effects appear to be worse for adolescent animals than adult animals. It also appears that the brain inflammation in the hippocampus caused by junk foods is more pronounced in juveniles, which highlights the increased vulnerability of the brain during early life. We'll discuss the hippocampus in more detail in Chapter 8, but suffice to say, junk food may be bad news for the developing adolescent brain.

Psychotic disorders

We've looked at the science and established that both mothers' and fathers' metabolic health (body weight, diabetes and high blood pressure) are linked to the risk for neurodevelopmental problems, such as ASD and ADHD and intellectual disability. But what about psychotic disorders, such as schizophrenia, which also have an important neurodevelopmental component?

First, based on the observational evidence, mothers with type 2 diabetes are more likely to have children who go on to develop schizophrenia. Large studies from Finland, the United States and Japan have also shown that the children of mothers who were obese before or during pregnancy were two to three times more likely to have schizophrenia. The studies in this area haven't necessarily taken into account a range of other factors that may have influenced the risk of those children developing schizophrenia, such as birth complications including emergency caesareans, placental abruption (separation of the placenta from the womb before birth) and perinatal asphyxia (lack of oxygen before, during or after birth). Each of these is associated with an increased risk of schizophrenia in children and is also more common in mothers with metabolic disorders, particularly obesity. Obese women are twice as likely to give birth via emergency caesarean section than mothers of normal weight. This all means that we have to be careful when assuming that one thing causes another. The data about schizophrenia are consistent, however, with what we know about other mental and brain disorders.

INFLAMMATION: AN IMPORTANT CONCEPT

Inflammation is the body's appropriate response to either injury or infection. If you have a gash in your leg or catch the flu, your immune system springs into action to heal the injury or fight off the virus or infection. The body creates a range of chemicals needed for these processes to occur and, as part of an acute (sudden-onset) response, these are entirely necessary for healing. Many aspects of our environment, health behaviours or health status can, however, cause a chronic (long-term), low-grade activation of the immune system, resulting in us being exposed to these inflammatory molecules for an extended period of time. This chronic systemic (body-wide) inflammation can increase the risk of a range of diseases, including heart disease and depression.

It won't surprise you to learn that unhealthy diets, as well as elevated blood glucose and obesity, are potent risk factors for inflammation, as well as for 'oxidative stress', which occurs when the body's antioxidant defences can't adequately

---

counteract the damaging effects of reactive oxygen species (free radicals). These two go together and each one is prompted by the other.

Inflammation and oxidative stress in both the mother and the fetus can have a range of harmful consequences, including reducing the levels of the omega-3 fatty acids that are so important for neurodevelopment, as well as of other nutrients such as iron and zinc. There is also 'neuroinflammation', which is simply inflammation in the brain. While the molecules used by the immune system are important in prompting and controlling aspects of brain development, abnormal levels can result in problems.

There's also evidence that when a mother contracts certain infections during vulnerable periods in her pregnancy – for example, influenza, rubella, polio, measles, herpes simplex, pneumonia and even tonsillitis – this can increase the risk of schizophrenia in the child. This increased risk, although small, can interact with pre-existing risk factors, such as a genetic inheritance, as well as with risk factors later in life. This is another important way that diet before and during pregnancy could influence the risk of mental disorders less directly, through a detrimental influence on the mothers' immune system. If mothers have an unhealthy diet, with or without obesity or diabetes, they may be less able to fight off the viruses or infections they're exposed to during pregnancy.

Food sensitivities, ASD and ADHD

For many years, the idea of removing gluten and/or dairy foods from the diets of children with ASD has been popular within the general public, particularly as children with ASD often suffer from gut problems. But although there's some limited evidence that children with ASD are more likely to have a sensitivity to cow's milk, there's no clear link between gluten sensitivity or coeliac disease and ASD. A review of the (pretty limited) research evidence concluded that overall rates of food allergy aren't higher in children with ASD than in those without.

While a number of intervention studies have attempted to show that removing these types of foods or food components from the diet is beneficial, the evidence so far is not very strong. Many (although not all) of the studies are poor quality and, so far, researchers who have considered all the data have concluded that there's no real benefit unless the child shows overt reactions to a particular food, in which case a more serious illness, such as coeliac disease, should be considered. Before removing such foods from a child's diet, it's important to obtain a proper diagnosis from a qualified medical practitioner who has assessed food sensitivities and allergies in the child using proper strategies (i.e. skin-prick testing, strict exclusion diets and food challenges). Whole dairy foods (not processed flavoured milks and yoghurts and processed cheeses, but whole milk, quality cheese and unsweetened yoghurts) and whole grains are very important sources of nutrients and fibre and removing these can reduce the quality of a child's diet. Not to mention the extra concern and effort and – often – expense involved in trying to avoid these foods.

Similarly, while children with allergic diseases such as eczema and asthma are more likely to develop ADHD, and children with ADHD are more at risk of allergic diseases, there's little evidence to suggest that children with ADHD have more food allergies than those without. There hasn't been much in the way of experiments to assess whether removing allergenic foods such as dairy, eggs and peanuts might be helpful, so it's impossible to say at this stage.

On the other hand, there is some evidence that around 10 per cent of children with ADHD respond quite strongly – with increased hyperactivity – when given food colourings and preservatives in controlled intervention studies. Given that these are found predominantly in processed foods, this presents another good reason to avoid them in your child's diet.

When it comes to psychotic illnesses (including bipolar disorder), there are a few anecdotal and case reports of people experiencing improvements when they remove grains or dairy from their diets. There's also evidence from research studies that people with psychotic illnesses have increased antibodies to gliadin, a protein found in grains (and that forms part of gluten). I suspect that a percentage of people with psychotic illnesses have food sensitivities or allergies that may exacerbate (not cause) their symptoms, but this needs more research to establish. This is another question that we at the Food & Mood Centre hope to investigate in the coming years.

It's also important to note that gut problems are very common in people with psychotic illnesses. Indeed, one autopsy study found evidence of gut damage in more than 90 per cent of people with schizophrenia. It's not clear, however, whether this is cause or consequence of the illness, and it's something we and other researchers are investigating to understand better.

Ketogenic diets

A number of case reports now suggest that a ketogenic diet may be helpful for some people with schizophrenia. In very simple terms, the ketogenic diet aims to remove nearly all carbohydrates (that is grains, rice, fruits, starchy vegetables and anything with sugar) from the diet and to ensure that the majority of calories come from fat. This very strict and limited diet has long been established as a useful treatment for children with epilepsy and seeks to make sure that the energy the brain uses comes from ketones from the breakdown of fats rather than glucose from the breakdown of carbohydrates. We'll talk about this in more detail in Chapter 11, but at this stage we can't say whether the benefits reported in a handful of people with schizophrenia were due to the ketogenic diet itself, or because these people removed foods (such as refined grains) they may have been allergic or sensitive to.

When Australian neuroscientists mimicked the symptoms of schizophrenia in mice then performed experiments on them, their results suggested that a ketogenic diet might be useful for symptoms of schizophrenia, just as it is for epilepsy. For this reason, our team is about to start a pilot study of this diet in people who are in hospital with psychotic illnesses, to see whether it might improve their symptoms. Unlike a traditional ketogenic diet, which prioritises animal foods and fats, we'll use a modified form that emphasises monounsaturated and polyunsaturated fats from avocados, nuts, fish and olive oil. Until we have the evidence from such studies, however, we would definitely not recommend such a diet, as it's extremely strict and demanding and requires close medical supervision. It also removes very important nutrients and fibre from the diet, which is likely to have a detrimental impact on the gut microbiota. High-fat diets can also result in a host of gut issues, as we'll see in more detail in Chapter 8.

Finally, because people with schizophrenia have altered glucose metabolism, which is exacerbated by the antipsychotic medications, they more commonly suffer from obesity, type 2 diabetes and other metabolic diseases. For this reason, many studies have investigated the impact of dietary and exercise programs for people with schizophrenia, with varying levels of success.

Our colleagues in Sydney have pioneered a successful lifestyle program for people with serious mental illnesses, showing that weight gain and metabolic illness can be largely avoided if the sufferers are supported to improve their diet and increase their exercise. This is an extremely important insight, as people with schizophrenia, on average, have a substantially shortened lifespan compared to the general population. To date, however, no studies have tried to assess whether such programs improve psychiatric symptoms and functioning. Such studies are not far away, however, so we watch this space with interest.

Key facts

- The quality of mothers' diets during pregnancy and children's diets in the first years of life are linked to children's emotional health *and* cognitive (brain) health.
- Omega-3 fatty acids from seafood are important for brain development from the start of life.
- Mothers' metabolic health (e.g. body weight, blood glucose, presence of metabolic syndrome) both before and during pregnancy is linked to their children's risk of autism, ADHD, cognitive delay and schizophrenia, as well as a range of congenital abnormalities.
- Fathers who are overweight or obese are more likely to have children with ASD.
- The reward systems of adolescents' brains are more receptive than those of adults, which may make junk food more enticing for them.
- Too much junk food may impair cognitive functioning and impulse control in adolescents.

- While a small percentage of children with ADHD respond to food colourings with increased hyperactivity, there's currently insufficient scientific evidence for excluding gluten or dairy from the diets of children with ADHD or ASD, or in people with psychotic illnesses.

7

Ageing well

My beloved mum is nearly 98 years old. She lives in a nursing home where she beams at everyone, talks to the remote control and eats her very regular meals and snacks with gusto. She seems happy and the carers tell me she's the only resident who doesn't complain and always gives a big smile to whoever is in her vicinity. But she's also completely incontinent, unable to walk, and has quite advanced dementia. She still recognises me, though, and I love to visit her to hold her hand, stroke her hair and listen to her chat – even though she doesn't make a lot of sense these days.

It wasn't always like this, of course. Mum was exceptionally bright until around the age of 93, with a quick wit, keen insight, and a robust and positive attitude. She'd had a very hard life, coming on the boat from the United Kingdom at the age of six with her large family; she was one of the original 'ten-pound Poms' who migrated to Australia after the Second World War. She, along with her parents, brothers and sisters, moved out to

Australia for a better life. My grandfather's brother had come earlier – leaving the cold, damp poverty of Birmingham to set up a sweets factory in Melbourne where he began to make a very good living. Fred had written to Grandad and said, 'Sell the shirt off your back and get over here – the sun shines!' They all made the long, rough sea journey and settled in to life in Australia, living together in my great-uncle's shed with its dirt floor. My grandad went to work cleaning railway carriages and mum went to school, although not for long. Like many of her generation, she left school at 12 and went to work in her uncle's factory, cleaning toilets and setting rat-traps. She always worked exceptionally hard, particularly after she became a single parent and needed to work as well as look after three children (my older half-brothers and sister). She worked in many different jobs, moving from factory to clerical work over the years. But she always had that robust and positive attitude and a strong constitution. Over the years her siblings gradually died, until she was the only one left. And still she lives, although her light is growing dimmer.

Why has she lived so long? What factors allowed her to maintain her cognitive faculties into her nineties? Clearly there must be a genetic factor there. One of her other siblings lived until 93 and another into his late eighties. Her father also lived a long life until he – possibly quite sensibly – decided, with a cup of tea and some sleeping tablets, to give up the business of living at 93. Mum's positive and sunny attitude no doubt helped things, but she also had a relatively good diet all her life. Like many of her generation, she ate simple food: porridge for breakfast, sandwiches with salad for lunch (she loved tinned salmon on sourdough rye toast), meat and vegetables for dinner, lots of cups of tea and the occasional biscuit. Many of her jobs involved physical labour, although that wasn't true later in her life.

Did her diet help her to stay cognitively well? It's not possible to know, but the evidence suggests that it might have. While we have to rely mainly on observational studies, with their methodological limitations and challenges, a growing body of evidence suggests that diet quality throughout life also influences our risk of cognitive decline and dementia.

Diet and dementia risk

Many studies have shown that people who have a more Mediterranean-style diet have a reduced risk of Alzheimer's disease and cognitive decline. In several studies of older US Americans, for example, higher intakes of vegetables, fruits, legumes, wholegrain cereals, fish and olive oil, lower intakes of meat and dairy foods, and moderate red wine consumption, were associated with a reduced risk of not only cognitive decline, but also Alzheimer's disease itself *and* with the risk of death. In a study of more than 1400 older people in Europe, higher adherence to a Mediterranean diet was associated with slower rates of cognitive decline over approximately five years. Similarly, an Australian study of more than 500 healthy older adults showed that higher scores on an Australian version of a Mediterranean-style dietary pattern were linked to lower rates of decline in aspects of cognitive functioning over a three-year period, while higher scores on a typical Western dietary pattern (red and processed meats, refined grains, chips, pizza, sweets and burgers) showed the opposite. Bringing all the data together, a large meta-analysis in 2013 concluded that a Mediterranean dietary pattern was associated with an approximate 40 per cent reduction in the risk of cognitive impairment. It's notable that it also found a reduced risk of depression and stroke associated with this style of diet.

Interestingly, in the Australian study that found an Australian-style of Mediterranean diet was related to better cognitive health outcomes, a healthy dietary pattern – which differed from the Mediterranean-style dietary pattern mainly with regard to fish intake – was not associated with improved measures of cognitive health. This suggests that fish intake may be particularly important in protecting the brain during the ageing process. Neuroinflammation in the brain is prompted by the amyloid-beta proteins that are a key feature of the plaques that form in Alzheimer's disease, and the anti-inflammatory omega-3 fatty acids in seafood may help counteract their impact. New evidence also shows that a protein (beta-parvalbumin) abundant in many types of fish, including cod, carp, redfish and herring, protects against the formation of amyloid proteins. This may be another way that fish can protect against dementia.

On the other hand, another study of roughly 400 older Scottish people showed that while lower adherence to a Mediterranean-style diet was associated with greater brain atrophy over a three-year period, this didn't seem to be explained by fish intake. Other fats in the diet are also relevant to brain health – high saturated fat, for example, appears to increase the risk of cognitive decline, while higher intakes of monounsaturated fats, found in olive oil, avocados and nuts, are protective. In a meta-analysis of studies examining food consumption in 11 countries around the globe, the higher fat levels in the food supply, and the higher the average energy consumption, the greater the prevalence of Alzheimer's disease, although this study could not differentiate between different types of fats. However, in another very recent meta-analysis, higher intakes of saturated fat were associated with an increased risk of Alzheimer's disease and dementia, while there was no observed association with other types of fats and dementia risk.

Many other studies have shown a link between higher saturated-fat intake and poorer measures of brain health, including reduced mental speed, flexibility, memory and verbal fluency. As a Mediterranean diet is low in saturated fats from animals, and high in mono- and polyunsaturated fats, this could be one of its key benefits. And, of course, a multitude of other components of a Mediterranean diet are likely to be protective of the brain, such as fibre, polyphenols and many other plant-based compounds. Another recent study showed that, over a span of three years, middle-aged people (30–60 years old) who had low adherence to a Mediterranean-style diet showed greater Alzheimer's plaque deposition and reductions in brain activity than people who had higher adherence. This suggests that diet has an impact on brain health and the risk of dementia well before old age.

While not all studies have shown a link between a Mediterranean-style diet and cognitive decline and dementia, we believe that the discrepancies are likely a result of the challenges of accurately recording and analysing dietary intakes. It's also true that many other lifestyle factors, such physical activity, alcohol consumption, smoking, education, social support, and – of course – genetic risk, are involved in the risk of cognitive decline and dementia. Teasing apart the contribution of each of these factors, alongside diet, is obviously challenging. For this reason, it's important that we also consider intervention studies, where diet has been manipulated and the impact on cognitive health measured.

The PREDIMED study

The PREDIMED (Prevención con Dieta Mediterránea) study was the largest dietary intervention (experiment) undertaken anywhere in the world. Because a lot of findings from this study tell us about the importance of diet for mental and brain health, I'll go into a bit of detail here. We'll be referring to this study again in Chapter 9.

PREDIMED recruited nearly 7500 European adults, aged between 55 and 80, who had risk factors for heart disease, such as type 2 diabetes, smoking, overweight or obesity, cholesterol problems, and/or a family history of heart disease. At the start of the study these people were randomly assigned to one of three diets: a Mediterranean diet where they were encouraged to consume at least 50 grams of good-quality, extra virgin olive oil every day; or a Mediterranean diet supplemented with a handful of raw mixed nuts every day (15 grams walnuts, 7.5 grams hazelnuts and 7.5 grams almonds); or a low-fat diet based on the dietary recommendations from the American Heart Association.

This low-fat diet was the 'control' (comparison) diet and, while it also included recommendations for increasing fruit and vegetable intake and reducing commercial baked goods, sweets and pastries, red and processed fatty meats, it also discouraged the consumption of olive oil, oily fats and nuts (in other words, sources of healthy fats).

The participants in PREDIMED all received individual and group-based support from dietitians to make the necessary changes to their diets over the period of the trial. The study ran for approximately five years and was stopped when it was clear that the people in both of the Mediterranean diet groups, compared to the ones in the low-fat diet group, were approximately 30 per cent less likely to have suffered a cardiac event in that time frame. They were also less likely to have metabolic syndrome, and their blood pressure, cholesterol, arteriosclerosis (hardening of the arteries), inflammation and oxidative stress were also improved compared to the low-fat group.

While cardiac events were the main outcome of interest in this study, many other results have come out of PREDIMED. One of these substudies that is relevant to this chapter, assessed a range of higher level cognitive abilities in some of the PREDIMED participants who participated in the study for a bit longer (6.5 years) than the main group. The researchers wanted to understand if there was an impact of the three types of diets on cognitive functioning. It won't surprise you to know that people in each of the two Mediterranean diet groups performed better on the measures of cognitive functioning at the end of the study than those in the low-fat-diet group.

Now the PREDIMED study wasn't perfect. Being the largest randomised controlled dietary trial (intervention study), it involved many logistical challenges and two of the 11 study sites didn't adhere properly to their randomisation protocol, meaning that at those two sites we can't be sure that any health effects were a result of the diets of the participants. This caused a bit of a fuss when it was discovered just recently, but when the study results were recalculated taking this into account, the main results didn't change. The limitations inherent in pretty much every scientific study means that we need to look at the weight of evidence from many different studies and not hang too much on just one study. Luckily, of course, there have been many studies of the Mediterranean diet and the results are pretty consistent in showing that it's a particularly healthy dietary pattern.

The PREDIMED study also had many important strengths, one of which was the length of time over which it was conducted. Investigating the possible impact of dietary change on brain health over a long enough time period is important, as it's more likely that changes in cognitive functioning can be observed. Another study that implemented a 'brain preservation' diet in elderly Chinese people, recommending two fruit and three leafy green vegetable portions a day, five fish servings per week and salt reduction, didn't show any improvements in cognitive functioning, but this study ran for less than three years. In line with this, a review of the evidence from short-term dietary experiments yields mixed results. This is mainly, I suspect, because short-term changes to diet are not easily reflected in the various measures of cognitive function that are assessed in these types of intervention studies.

Even in short-term intervention studies, however, there's fairly consistent evidence that energy restriction (that is, reducing the number of calories eaten) can benefit working memory – the memory we use to keep information in our minds while we perform complex tasks. Lowering energy intake and reducing fat consumption or moving fat consumption from saturated to mono- and polyunsaturated fats, also seems to be beneficial to long-term memory, particularly in people who are overweight or obese. It also appears to benefit executive functioning, which is the most complex of the cognitive domains and concerns the ability to adapt in a positive way to situations using problem-solving, mental flexibility and planning. Various studies have also shown that reducing saturated fat and increasing mono- and polyunsaturated fats improves visual-spatial memory, which helps us to record information about our environment and its spatial orientation.

Cardiometabolic health and dementia risk

Because of the challenges in assessing long-term dietary habits, and of manipulating diet and measuring its effect on brain function in both the short and long term, it's important to understand that more exact measures of health, such as obesity, high insulin and insulin resistance, type 2 diabetes, high blood pressure and high cholesterol, are all risk factors for dementia and cognitive decline. Of course, these cardiometabolic factors are also clearly influenced by dietary habits. Even raised blood glucose within the normal range (which is exceedingly common) is now established as a risk factor for dementia. Indeed, colleagues of mine showed that high blood glucose in the normal range was related to greater atrophy in key regions of the brain relevant to ageing and neurodegenerative processes – the hippocampus and the amygdala – in older Australians. High blood glucose results in reductions in levels of neurotransmitters, magnesium and B-group vitamins, but it also results in something else that has been recently identified as problematic to health: advanced glycation end products, or AGEs.

AGEs

AGEs are formed in our bodies when sugars are combined with amino acids (the building blocks of proteins) or fats in a process called 'glycation'. This means that if we have high blood glucose we'll produce more AGEs. Not only do we make our own AGEs, but we also get them directly from our diet. Meats, poultry and even fish, particularly when high in fat, are the major source of dietary AGEs. They are produced when these animal products are browned at high temperatures, such as during grilling, roasting, searing, frying and baking. Other sources of dietary AGEs are fatty junk foods such as pizza, hamburgers, commercial macaroni and cheese, and even toasted cheese sandwiches! Healthy foods don't all get off scot-free, though: roasting nuts also increases their AGE content. Dairy products and carbohydrate-rich plant foods, such as vegetables, fruits and grains, contain the least AGEs, even when cooked. Grain products cooked in dry heat, such as baked biscuits and crackers, do have some AGEs, but far less than is found in animal foods.

AGEs cause problems in cells by altering the function of proteins, and can 'clog' the microvascular system throughout the body. They also appear to increase systemic inflammation, which as we've already established is a risk factor for depression and heart disease, as well as for type 2 diabetes and Alzheimer's disease. The glycation of proteins results in much higher levels of oxidative stress, and oxidative stress can also cause more AGEs! Studies have reported higher concentrations of AGE-positive neurons and AGE antibodies in the hippocampal brain tissue of people who died with Alzheimer's disease than in people who died from other causes.

While there's still much we don't understand about AGEs and the research results are not always clear-cut (as just one example, high levels of AGEs are found in many healthy older people as well as those with disease), it's now believed that avoiding excessive AGEs may help to delay chronic disease and ageing. The evidence from both animal and human studies does suggest that that adopting a low-AGE diet can reduce systemic inflammation. The best approach to reducing AGEs is to use wet heat forms of cooking (steaming), slow-cooking at lower temperatures, and marinating animal foods in acids such as lemon or vinegar before cooking, which inhibits the formation of AGEs. Following a Mediterranean-style diet, which commonly uses such marinades and also limits fatty and processed meats, is a pretty good strategy for lowering AGEs.

How we can protect our brain health

If we bring all of the data together, it seems that the quality of our diets over our lifetime can influence our brain health and risk of developing dementia. It seems particularly important to eat lots of plant foods and healthy fats, such as those found in oily fish, olive oil, avocados and nuts, and to avoid foods that we know are detrimental to brain health, such as those with high levels of added sugars and both saturated and hydrogenated (trans) fats. By keeping a close eye on what we put in our mouths, as well as on our metabolic health (body weight, blood cholesterol, blood glucose and blood pressure), and remaining physically, mentally and socially active, we're more likely to live longer and happier lives.

Key facts

- Elevated blood glucose (even in the 'high normal' range), type 2 diabetes, obesity, high insulin and insulin resistance, high blood pressure and high cholesterol are all risk factors for dementia and cognitive decline.
- People eating Mediterranean-style diets have a reduced risk of Alzheimer's disease and cognitive decline.
- Both fish oils and fish proteins appear to protect the brain during the ageing process.
- High saturated fat intake appears to increase the risk of cognitive decline, while higher intakes of monounsaturated fats, found in olive oil, avocados and nuts, are protective.
- Reducing energy intake (that is, calories) seems to result in improvements in memory.
- High blood glucose, as well as the browning of foods by cooking at high temperatures (particularly animal foods), results in the formation of advanced glycation end products (AGEs). These are associated with chronic diseases and diseases of ageing, so avoiding these (using steaming, marinating and/or slow-cooking) may be beneficial to health.

8

The immune system, brain plasticity, epigenetics and gut microbiota in mental health

If you want to understand the mechanisms behind the link between diet and mental and brain health, read on. This chapter is a bit technical in parts, so you can skip it if you're not particularly interested in how the car works but are happy just to drive it!

The immune system: your inner Viking and the key to health

People used to think that mental disorders only existed in our head and that there was a clear distinction between our minds and bodies. But now we increasingly understand that we're one highly complex system and that there can and should be no real separation.

We already took a brief look at systemic inflammation in the previous chapter. This occurs when the immune system, instead of being activated in the short term to help you heal from an injury or an infection, is switched onto 'low' and stays there. The resulting molecules that circulate throughout the body help to drive the inflammatory process and can increase the risk of many diseases, including heart disease and obesity.

One of the key insights that started to change the way we think about the connection between physical and mental health was the evidence that inflammation may also play a part in prompting depression, as well as being affected by both stress and depressive illness. How did this understanding come about?

The first clues were the fact that immune function is often impaired in people who are experiencing stress. You would recognise this in your own life – stressful periods often seem to result in a virus or some sort of illness, and we've all had the very annoying experience of falling sick on the first day of our holidays! I know that my immune function goes right down when I'm stressed. What I particularly notice is that my gums start to get sore and to bleed more easily. When I asked my dentist why I would get gingivitis when I have good oral hygiene, his first question was, 'Are you stressed?' He says that in his practice he sees a very clear link between stress and gum disease. This is particularly interesting to me, because of our research interest in the microbiota that live in our mouths as well as in our gut. It seems that they may be some sort of barometer of health; I certainly know to pay attention to my stress levels when my gums start to bleed.

Stress activates a range of neurotransmitter pathways as well as the stress-response system. These systems, in turn, influence many important components of the immune system, including the lymph organs, spleen, bone marrow, thymus gland and gut, while the immune system itself acts upon the stress-response system in a bidirectional relationship. What it basically means is that when we're stressed, our immune system doesn't work as well. The stress response also prompts neuroinflammation – inflammation in the brain. Stress, of course, is also one of many important risk factors for depression.

The next pieces of evidence come from studies in people with clinical depression. When we have an infection or injury, hormones called cytokines are released. These act as the messengers of the immune system and activate our immune responses. These inflammatory markers, as well as others such as C-reactive protein (CRP), are higher in the blood of many people suffering from depression. Markers of oxidative stress, which goes along with inflammation, are also higher. There's also intriguing data showing that nutrient levels such as zinc can be lower in people with depression (regardless of their diet), but that they return to a higher level once those people recover from their depressive episode (without taking any supplements). Zinc, folate, and other nutrients are lowered as a result of biochemical changes that occur when the stress and immune systems are activated. In other words, lower levels of nutrients in the blood might be a result of mental illness itself.

In many people with depression, levels of long-chain omega-3 fatty acids are also lower, and this is thought to be at least partly due to the increased oxidative stress that goes along with the inflammation. The membranes of the neurons in the brain and other cells are primarily made up of fatty acids, and they are vulnerable to oxidative damage from free radicals. Inflammation 'burns up' the important omega-3 fatty acids, reducing their levels in our body and brain.

The third piece of evidence comes from animal experiments. When cytokines are administered to rodents they cause what is known as 'sickness behaviour'. Animals are no different from humans in that they behave differently when they're sick. They're less active and spend more time sleeping, they lose their appetite and groom themselves less, they limit their social interactions with other rodents, and seem less interested in what's going on around them. This sickness behaviour is thought to be so similar to depression in humans that it's regarded as an animal model of depression.

Importantly, when a cytokine (specifically interferon alpha) is given as a treatment for some cancers and viral infections in humans, it also induces depression, cognitive impairment and reduced motivation in many of these people. Interestingly, antidepressant medications appear to dampen down inflammation by reducing the production of 'pro-inflammatory' cytokines and increasing the production of 'anti-inflammatory' cytokines, although this mechanism appears to be impaired in people with serious depression.

Finally, our team has also produced observational evidence from the Geelong Osteoporosis Study (GOS) to suggest that systemic inflammation, indicated by raised inflammatory markers (in this case, CRP) in the blood, increases the risk of major depressive disorder. We measured women's CRP at the start of the study and then followed them for ten years, noting whether they developed major depression during that time. We saw that women with higher levels of CRP at the start were more likely to develop major depression in a dose–response manner. That is, the higher their CRP (inflammation) at the start of the study, the higher their risk of clinical depression over time.

For all these reasons, many researchers now believe that systemic inflammation is both a cause and a consequence of depressive disorders. But what causes the inflammation? Well, many aspects of our modern lives, including stress, low vitamin D levels, insufficient sleep, insufficient exercise, poor dental health and gum disease, allergies, smoking and obesity. But at this point in the book, it won't surprise you to learn that one of the key contributors to systemic inflammation is a Western diet.

Diet and inflammation

Many studies tell us that diet quality has an important impact on inflammation. For example, in the large Nurses' Health Study in the United States, which tracked nearly 45,000 women, those with a healthier dietary pattern, with higher intakes of vegetables and fruit, whole grains, fish and legumes, had lower levels of CRP and pro-inflammatory cytokines. In contrast, in both this study and another large study in men, an unhealthy ('Western') dietary pattern, high in red and processed meats, refined carbo-hydrates and other processed foods, was associated with increased inflammatory markers. People who eat Mediterranean-style diets also have lower levels of inflammation.

Numerous studies now measure the 'inflammatory potential' of diet using a dietary inflammatory index (DII). In these studies, higher scores on a DII – meaning that the diet has more of the foods associated with raised inflammatory markers – is linked to an increased risk of depression. Again in the large Nurses' Health Study, higher DII scores were associated with an approximate 40 per cent increased risk of developing depression over 12 years of follow-up. This inflammatory dietary pattern had higher intakes of both sugar-sweetened and artificially sweetened fizzy drinks, red and processed meats, and refined grains (e.g. white flour), but was low in wine, coffee, olive oil, green leafy and other vegetables. In other words, the opposite of a Mediterranean dietary pattern. My colleagues and I have recently published a meta-analysis of diet quality, measured with many different types of dietary indices, and depression risk and we see – consistent with all the other data – that people with the lowest scores on an inflammatory dietary pattern are about 30% less likely on average to develop depression.

Aspects of many healthy and Mediterranean-style diets appear to especially influence inflammation. For example, the fibre in wholegrain foods – an important part of a Mediterranean diet – appears to be particularly beneficial to the immune system; wholegrain foods are rich in beta-glucans, which are known to promote immune function. Wholegrain foods are also high in phytochemicals, which protect against the oxidative stress that is a consequence of inflammation and a feature of depressive illness. It's notable that a particularly huge meta-analysis of more than 300 meta-analyses (yep, a meta-analysis of meta-analyses), breaking down everything we know about diet and health from the observational literature, found that the consumption of whole grains was the most protective against diet-related chronic diseases – even more so than fruits and vegetables! Our very new, yet rapidly developing, understanding of the importance of the bacteria that live in our gut – and its reliance on dietary fibre – is providing a new perspective on whole grains, which we'll cover in more detail later in this chapter.

High-glycemic-load (GL) diets are a common feature of Western culture, and are heavy in refined carbohydrates (white breads, rice, processed cereals) and added sugars. High-GL diets are consistently associated with higher levels of CRP. Similarly, diets high in omega-6 fatty acids, which are commonly used in the production of processed foods (refined seed and soybean oils), increase the production of pro-inflammatory cytokines, while omega-3 fatty acids, which are important components of many healthy foods, such as seafood, nuts, legumes and leafy green vegetables, have potent anti-inflammatory effects. As I mentioned earlier, we in the West don't eat enough of these omega-3s. Saturated fats (found in animal foods) are also linked to inflammation in humans: in the large British Whitehall II cohort study, higher levels of saturated fatty acids in the blood were associated with higher CRP, while higher polyunsaturated fatty acid levels were associated with lower CRP levels.

Many intervention trials in humans also show that a change in diet can change inflammation status. In one study, when overweight people were put on a sugar-rich diet for ten weeks, this resulted in increased inflammation. I'm not quite sure if we'd get ethics approval to do that these days, given what we now know about the damaging effects of sugar! I'm betting those participants didn't feel so great after ten weeks of a high-sugar diet.

There's also evidence that we can improve our inflammatory status by increasing our healthy food intake. In one study, for example, men who were put on a diet high in fruits and vege-tables (eight serves per day) for eight weeks showed a significant decrease in inflammation compared to those eating only two serves per day.

Imagine how that might look for you in your daily diet. How might you get all those fruits and vegetables into your meals?

Improving our diet for good health: a practical example

Let's think about a day in the diet of a typical Australian bloke. Breakfast might be a processed cereal, made with refined wheat and with a lot of added sugar. The packet might say something like 'made with whole grains', or 'low in fat', but a quick read of the label would tell you that the sugar content was high and the main ingredient was white flour (maybe with some salt, emulsifiers and other chemicals thrown in for good luck). Or he might have some white-bread toast with margarine and jam, along with a big glass of orange juice, or some eggs, sausages and bacon with toast. Morning tea might be a pastry or biscuit with a cup of coffee. Lunch could be a white bread roll with chicken schnitzel (perhaps without the lettuce) and some mayonnaise, with another sweet drink (maybe flavoured milk or a fizzy drink). Or maybe a bucket of hot chips with a pie and a soft drink. Afternoon tea might be another sweet treat of some sort, and dinner might be some sausages with a couple of vegetables, with another couple of slices of white bread. Or maybe it would be takeaway from a well-known 'food' chain involving fried chicken or similar, with a sad little lettuce leaf and slice of tomato on the side. Or even just pasta with a vegie-free bolognese sauce. There would be ice cream or cake for dessert, followed by some couch snacks to see him through until bedtime.

Do you see the problem? That diet would exceed, many times over, the recommendations for sugar intake. It would also be full of the wrong sorts of fats, too much salt, and most likely artificial sugars and emulsifiers – all a disaster for his gut and his brain. Critically, it would also be almost entirely lacking in all the multitudes of vitamins, minerals, polyphenols, fibre and healthy fats that we know are so important for the functioning of the body and brain.

We know what the likely result of this diet would be. This poor bloke would get to 50 or so and likely be overweight or obese. His doctor might also have told him that he needed medications for high blood pressure and high cholesterol. His blood glucose would be high, and he might even be diabetic. And his inflammatory markers would be high. What would this mean? A very real likelihood that he would not make old bones. Heart attacks, stroke, cancer and diabetes all follow this sort of trajectory. This man would be less likely to see his grandchildren grow up, and even if he was lucky enough to survive into his seventies, he would be rattling like a pillbox and feeling far less than full of vigour and verve. And then, of course, his cognitive faculties could also take a hit, and the first signs of dementia would set in.

Let's see how we might turn this around: breakfast might be porridge instead of sweetened breakfast cereal. Or even unsweetened muesli. Sliced apple and banana would give him two serves of fruit, and the whole grains would provide essential fibre for his immune system. He could add a bit of honey if he needed the sweetness kick. Morning tea might be a couple of baby carrots with some hummus, brought from home. I live on baby carrots, and hummus is possibly my favourite food. Because it's made with chickpeas and tahini, it's very high in fibre and healthy fats and makes everything taste great. It counts towards your vegetable tally as well. Lunch might be a wholegrain roll with different sorts of salad vegetables: tomatoes, mixed lettuce, onion, grated carrot and beetroot, topped off with some tinned tuna. He could add some grated cheese for flavour. Drinks could be water, tea, coffee, coconut water, or even kombucha if he was feeling very adventurous! Afternoon tea can a big handful of raw nuts along with another piece of fruit. And that pasta bolognese for dinner? He could add chopped and grated vegetables to the sauce – carrots or sweet potatoes, zucchini, fresh tomatoes, mushrooms, leafy greens, as well as onion and garlic. He could tip in a tin of chickpeas or lentils as well – for more fibre. Then add a slice of wholegrain sourdough bread or replace the white pasta with wholemeal, spelt or buckwheat pasta (all available from the supermarket). Dessert could be my favourite – whole Greek yoghurt with frozen berries. He could put some honey on top if he really needed sweetness.

Maybe add a couple of dates – these are really sweet and are full of fibre. He could even have a couple of pieces of dark chocolate, full of polyphenols (just not the whole block).

There you have it. He's exceeded his tally of fruit and vegetables and managed to get a whole lot of fibre, healthy fats and even some fermented foods in to boot. Keep that up and he'd lose weight, reduce his inflammation and his risk of a whole host of diseases. He might even start to feel a lot more energetic, clear-headed and happier!

There's more evidence from intervention studies: people on a diet high in soy, nuts and plant foods for a month showed pronounced reductions in CRP levels, quite independently of changes in body weight. Again, inflammatory markers were reduced when people with metabolic syndrome (high blood pressure, high blood glucose, excess abdominal fat and high cholesterol) were put on a Mediterranean-style diet, again quite independently of any decreases in weight. In fact, a systematic review and meta-analysis of all of the intervention studies using a Mediterranean diet as their 'treatment' concluded that a Mediterranean diet significantly improves all aspects of the metabolic syndrome, while another showed the same result for the Mediterranean diet in treating inflammation, with reductions in CRP, cytokines and other inflammatory markers.

Finally, many animal studies homing in on mechanisms of action have shown that rodents on diets high in saturated fats have elevated markers of brain inflammation compared to those receiving standard diets. Other studies point again to the importance of diet during pregnancy; rats born to mothers who had been fed a high-saturated-fat diet during pregnancy had increased markers of neuroinflammation, as well as impaired spatial memory. Other studies suggest that even a rodent that eats a standard diet after birth, will have higher neuroinflammation as an adult if its mother was fed a high-saturated-fat diet during pregnancy. Given that inflammatory events during pregnancy are related to an increased risk of neurodevelopmental problems in children, this suggests that diets high in saturated fats during pregnancy might affect brain health in offspring.

Can junk food reprogram the immune system?

A recent study found that mice fed a high-fat, high-sugar, low-fibre diet – similar to a Western diet – very quickly developed a strong immune response, as if fighting off a bacterial infection. The researchers found that the diet had activated a large number of genes in the bone marrow of the mice, making them produce many more inflammatory molecules. But what was really worrying was that even when the mice were put back on a normal diet for a month, the genetic reprogramming of the inflammatory response remained. In other words, the junk-food diet reprogrammed the immune system of the animals to continue to respond to even minor stimuli with a strong inflammatory response. This finding has important implications, given the key role of systemic inflammation in so many physical diseases as well as in mental and brain health.

Obesity and inflammation

Obesity, another consequence of a Western diet, is an inflammatory condition in itself. Inflammatory cytokines are found in abundance in fat cells, particularly in abdominal fat cells, and are released into the circulation. This is of particular relevance given the strong 'bidirectional' relationship between depression and obesity (meaning that one increases the risk of the other, and vice versa). People with clinical depression are at increased risk of weight gain, particularly around the abdomen, and this is thought to relate to the stress hormones that prompt the body to put on fat around the stomach. In other words, because of our stress hormones, a depressed person might gain more stomach fat than a non-depressed person even if their diet and exercise were the same. And obesity is also a risk factor for depression. This is believed to be at least partly a consequence of the cytokines released by fat cells. A recent meta-analysis concluded that obesity increases the risk of later depression by 55 per cent, while depression increases the risk of developing obesity by 58 per cent. The *good* news is, however, that losing weight off the belly can reduce cytokine levels.

EARLY LIFE EXPERIENCES AND INFLAMMATION

One important point about inflammation and depression is that people who were exposed to trauma in childhood appear to be particularly prone to systemic inflammation, which in turn increases their risk of all manner of chronic diseases, including depression. For example, a large study in New Zealand that followed 1000 children from birth to their thirties showed that those who had experienced maltreatment, abuse, social isolation and economic hardship during childhood were twice as likely to have chronic systemic inflammation. US researchers concluded that childhood adversity can *shorten the lifespan by seven to 15 years*, potentially as a consequence of increased inflammation and cell ageing. All of these findings point to the importance of reducing or avoiding the things that can chronically increase inflammation. And key among these is an unhealthy diet.

Brain plasticity

Until the 1980s, it was commonly believed that we lost brain neurons as we aged. But scientists then began to confirm, using animal studies, what some people had suspected since the 1960s – that regions of the brain appear to grow new brain cells all the time.

One of these areas that we know is particularly relevant to mental and brain health is the hippocampus. The hippocampus actually comprises two little structures, sitting side by side in the middle of the brain, that look a bit like seahorses. Hippocampus is the name of the genus to which seahorses belong; the name comes from the Greek words for 'horse' and 'sea monster'. The hippocampus, from what we understand so far (and of course our knowledge is increasing all the time), is key to our memory – particularly our long-term memory for facts and events. In other words, it's critical to our ability to learn and remember things. It's one of the first areas of the brain to show signs of damage in dementia.

The hippocampus also appears to be a key region involved in our emotional regulation and mental health. People with depression have a smaller hippocampus, while successful treatment with antidepressants results in the hippocampus growing again. In fact, prompting the growth of new brain cells in the hippocampus is one of the key ways antidepressants and other psychiatric medications seem to work. This shrinking and growing of the hippocampus, with a resulting impact on forms of memory and (we think) mental health, is called 'brain plasticity'.

One of the key factors that determines the growth of new neurons in the brain is a polypeptide called brain-derived neurotrophic factor, or BDNF. I think of BDNF as manure for the brain: it protects the existing neurons from oxidative stress and also promotes the growth of new neurons. Lower levels of

BDNF are seen in people with depression, bipolar disorder and schizophrenia, where the degree of shrinkage in the hippocampus is linked to the duration and severity of the illness. There has been much research into BDNF, and animal studies tell us that levels of BDNF and related brain plasticity are very quickly affected by many factors in our environment and our behaviour.

Stress is one key factor that reduces BDNF. Indeed, it's thought that a reduction in the growth of new neurons in the hippocampus as a result of stress may be an important trigger for depressive episodes, while the reversal of these changes and the restoration of healthy neuronal growth may help someone recover from an episode. Exercise is another key factor influencing brain plasticity. In fact, research evidence suggests that this is one main pathway by which exercise benefits our brain – it increases BDNF and other similar factors, which in turn increase the number of neurons in the hippocampus, as well as other types of brain cells (called astrocytes), and it also protects the brain against oxidative stress. Another new insight from science is that our muscles might give rise to BDNF – in other words, increasing our muscle power might also build our brain power! Intriguingly, in animals, social interactions and having an 'enriched environment' (that is, exercise wheels, things to explore, other animals in the cage and so on) seem to do this as well. You won't be surprised to learn, however, that diet is also a key factor influencing BDNF and brain plasticity.

Diet and brain plasticity

In animal experiments, many aspects of diet have a potent impact on BDNF, hippocampal neuron growth and function, and inflammatory processes in the brain that also affect the hippocampus. Food components such as omega-3 fatty acids, flavonoids, antioxidant-rich berries and resveratrol, a polyphenol found in red grapes and other fruits (and in red wine), stimulate the growth of new brain cells and reduce oxidative stress and pro-inflammatory processes. In contrast, high-fat and refined-sugar diets, as models of 'Western' diets, reduce the growth of new neurons, increase oxidative stress and promote inflammation, thus causing reductions in brain cells and problems with learning and memory. Long-term intake of such a diet causes cognitive deficits in animals, especially in memory tasks that require the hippocampus. Importantly, the longer an animal is exposed to these sorts of diets, the more profound the impact on their cognitive functioning and brain plasticity. Even a short spell on the high-fat and high-sugar diet results in cognitive impairments. A recent animal experiment showed that a diet rich in sugar and fat, or rich in sugar alone, resulted in impairments in hippocampal-dependent memory, independently of weight changes, in as little as five days.

Importantly, obese people – even children – show deficits in memory, learning and executive functions compared to people in the healthy weight range, although it's not clear whether it's obesity itself, poor diet, or a combination of both that contributes to the problem. In one of the few intervention studies with humans, sedentary but otherwise healthy men who ate a high-fat, ketogenic-style diet for one week performed worse on cognitive tasks than they had before the diet.

Does junk food shrink your brain?

On the basis of the animal studies looking at the impact of diet on brain plasticity, I was very keen to see whether the same sorts of associations would be true in humans. In 2014 I went to work with colleagues at the Australian National University in Canberra to investigate whether there was a link between dietary patterns and hippocampal size in humans, taking into account other factors that might explain any relationships we saw. This study took advantage of the data that had been collected from approximately 250 older Australians. My colleagues on this study had already demonstrated that higher blood glucose levels were linked to smaller hippocampal size in this cohort of people, but it wasn't clear if this was related to the quality of their diets.

We had already shown in a previous study that poor diet quality was linked to an increased risk of depression in these older people, and that healthier diets were linked to a reduced risk of depression, even when we factored in detailed measures of socioeconomic circumstances, such as income, education, employment and welfare status. Now, however, considering all of these factors *plus* depression, we wanted to directly test two hypotheses: that dietary patterns higher in nutrient- and antioxidant-rich foods would be associated with larger hippocampal volumes; and that dietary patterns higher in saturated fats and refined carbohydrates would be associated with smaller hippocampal volumes.

Again, it won't surprise you to learn that we found that both lower scores on a healthy dietary pattern and higher scores on an unhealthy dietary pattern were associated with smaller hippocampal size. We also found that – in common with a lot of the studies we'd conducted looking at mental health as the end point – diets high in junk and processed foods were associated with smaller hippocampal size, no matter the intake of healthy foods. And vice versa. In other words, both not getting enough of the good stuff and getting too much of the bad stuff were problematic. This was in line with our hypotheses, but what *was* somewhat surprising to us was the strength of the relationships.

Because we'd measured hippocampal size at two time points, four years apart, we could clearly see the reductions in hippocampal size that come with age ('age-related hippocampal atrophy'). This age-related shrinkage in our brain is a bit depressing and reinforces the importance of doing all we can to reduce this atrophy, including exercising, not smoking, keeping our brains active and keeping our social networks alive and healthy as we get older. But the quality of people's diets was equivalent to a large chunk of that age-related shrinkage (roughly 60 per cent) in our study.

As I write, a new, far larger study from the Netherlands has just been published showing that a healthier diet is associated with larger hippocampal volume – in line with what we observed – but also a larger total brain volume, grey matter volume and white matter volume. This study involved more than 4000 older adults who were free of dementia.

The main researcher on this study said to the press:

> There is much confusion around diet and brain health and it's up to doctors to provide clarity. One day people are told they should go vegan; the next day they can't touch bread.
>
> The scientific literature thus far indicates that a balanced diet pattern rich in healthy carbs and fibre, with low-to-moderate fat content, is supportive of brain aging. There is no evidence for the opposite, which provides a strong argument in favor of recommending a Mediterranean-style diet for brain aging and dementia prevention.

I agree.

Epigenetics

While stress plays an important role in the development of depression, it's clear that many people don't develop depression after serious stressful experiences, whereas other people can do so after experiencing even relatively minor stressful events. This highlights the importance of the interaction between the environment and our genes in the risk of depression. While some studies suggest that genetic factors account for as much as 40–50 per cent of the risk of developing depression, no specific genetic variants associated with depression have been reliably identified. There's some evidence for the involvement of genes related to neurotransmitter production and signalling and also BDNF (brain plasticity), but the results aren't consistent. This is probably due to the fact that depression is a complex, multifactorial disorder that is likely to involve many genes rather than just one.

New information that has come to light over the last couple of decades, however, has led us to understand that other important processes determine gene activity. One such process is epigenetics, which refers to the molecular marks that are deposited on our DNA or the proteins with which it's packaged in the cell (*epi* means 'on top of'). I work with a wonderful geneticist at Deakin, Professor Jeff Craig, who is a fantastic science communicator. He likens epigenetics to the musicians that play the 'symphony of life' on your genes.

Epigenetic codes drive our early development and are passed on every time a cell divides but can sometimes be changed by environment. Intriguingly, a small subset of epigenetic codes is also passed on to us from our parents, and possibly even our grandparents. This is why there's a new idea that you're not just what you eat, but what your grandparents ate. In other words, some environmental 'memories' are passed down and influence the activity of our genes. Twice per generation, most epigenetic memories are erased, but some remain to be passed on to subsequent generations. And it appears that these epigenetic memories can affect a range of outcomes, including brain development and functioning.

There are three key periods when epigenetic processes are 'registered': ancestral (our parents and even our grandparents), prenatally (i.e. during development) and postnatally. Of these, the prenatal period is by far the most important in terms of the impact on developmental and health outcomes. Many different exposures can influence epigenetic processes during development, including maternal age, substances use or abuse (alcohol, smoking, cocaine, cannabis), medications, infections, stress, pollutants and – of course – diet.

Although this field of research is in its infancy, there's growing evidence to suggest that aspects of diet, including folate, polyphenols, flavonoids and even caffeine, can affect epigenetic regulation 'globally' and on specific genes. Nutrients in the diet, such as folate (B_9), choline, methionine, betaine and methylcobalamin (B_{12}), are all particularly important in regulating epigenetic processes, so deficiencies in these important nutrients – particularly during pregnancy – may cause epigenetic alterations in developmental genes. In animal studies, feeding pregnant animals diets deficient in some of these key nutrients resulted in changes to genes that are essential for normal brain development and function in offspring. Some of these changes could be reversed by feeding the animals omega-3 fatty acids.

Other nutrients, such as zinc, selenium, iron, vitamins A and D and B vitamins, and polyphenols from plants have all been shown to affect the development of embryos by regulating epigenetic processes. Animal studies also show that high-fat diets during pregnancy can result in offspring with symptoms of metabolic syndrome, and this seems to arise from epigenetic alterations in genes important for the formation of fatty tissues in newborns.

It's also believed that epigenetic processes may be a pathway linking maternal type 2 diabetes to brain and other malformations in offspring. This is because the oxidative stress and inflammation that arise from too much glucose in the blood can disrupt the expression of many genes involved in the development of the fetus.

Inherited and epigenetic changes that are acquired *after* birth can also affect health – it's thought that epigenetic changes resulting from a range of environmental exposures (poor diet, smoking, stress and many others) can combine with genetic risk factors to reach a critical mass over time that 'tips the balance', resulting in disease. This may be relevant to psychotic illnesses such as schizophrenia, which don't usually manifest until late adolescence/early adulthood. While this field is still very young, the more we understand about how our diets can influence the way our genes work, the more we'll be able to target these processes to enhance and protect our health.

EPIGENETICS AND THE NEXT GENERATION

Let's return to the real world for a moment and think about the massively high rates of overweight and obesity we're now seeing in children. Then think about the quality of their daily diet, full of soft drinks, pizzas, chips, pies, hamburgers, doughnuts, ice creams, sausages, hot dogs, fried chicken, ham and bacon, and a myriad of other food products.

Then let's think about all the foods they're *not* eating: spinach, silverbeet, watercress, radicchio, parsley, broccoli, cauliflower, beetroot, sweet potato, lentils, chickpeas, green beans, peas, fish, apples, plums, berries, pears, oats, rye, barley, brown rice, whole wheat, olive oil, avocados, almonds, walnuts, cashews, brazil nuts . . . the list goes on and on. Then let's consider the essential elements found in those foods – the many, many active compounds, antioxidants, vitamins, minerals, polyphenols, healthy fats, fibre and all the other parts of whole foods that go towards running the incredibly awe-inspiring system that is the human body.

Now think, is my child or are the children I know going to be able to create healthy babies when the time comes for them to have a family? Are they going to have a healthy body weight? Low blood sugar? Low levels of inflammation? High levels of all those essential nutrients needed for the 'right' epigenetic marks? Are they going to have good eating habits they can pass on to their children? Do they know how to shop for fresh foods and prepare them?

These are the questions we need to ask ourselves and think about for the sake of future generations of children. We're at a crisis point, as our upcoming discussion of the human microbiota will bring into even sharper relief.

The gut and its resident microbiota

We're covered in bugs. In fact, we have trillions of different microorganisms living both on us and within us. They live in our mouths, on our skin, in our vagina if we're female, in our gut, and in every nook and cranny of the human body. Astoundingly, 99.5 per cent of our genes aren't even human; they're microbial. At least half of our cells are microbial! So, in some important sense, we're really more bug than human.

We didn't know much about the role of these microorganisms in our health until relatively recently as we didn't have the specialised tools and techniques needed to investigate them properly. But now, since developing new gene-sequencing technologies, we know that these 'commensal' bacteria (living with us and off us, without causing us harm) co-evolved with us and are a major player in our body's processes. In fact, we can't live without them and they can't live without us.

The largest number of these microbes live in our gut. In fact, the community of bacteria and their genetic material living in the gut is estimated to number roughly 100 trillion. The weight of the microbes in our gut is approximately the same as the weight of our brain. Indeed, some people refer to the gut micro-biota as our 'second brain'. This is because our gut has its own nervous system that works quite independently of our central nervous system. While we've known for a long time that our gut and brain are very closely connected and that they talk to each other all the time, we've only recently understood that the microbes that live *in* our gut are also profoundly important. From what we know so far, the gut and its resident microbes play a critical role in our immune functioning, metabolism, body weight and brain health, and possibly even in our behaviour.

But before we address that in detail, let's take a quick look at what we know so far about what microbiota – gut microbiota in particular – actually *do*.

From one end to another: a trip down the alimentary canal

When we take a bite of food, we chomp it up in our mouth and turn it into slush, which then makes its way down to the stomach where it's broken down further, before the slush (called chyme by this stage) proceeds to the small intestine. Which is actually not very small at all; it's approximately 6 metres long and – with all its nooks, crannies, and projections (called villi) – has a surface area of about 37 square metres. This ensures plenty of opportunity for water, salt and nutrients, including simple sugars and fats, to be absorbed directly into our system. There are plenty of bacteria in our small intestine, and some of them – like those from the *Bilophila* genus – do very well when we eat saturated fats, such as those found in bacon and sausages. Saturated fats prompt the release of bile from our liver and gallbladder, and *Bilophila* quite like this bile. The problem is that the *Bilophila* bacteria aren't the ones we want to encourage; they can trigger inflammation and are associated with a range of inflammatory diseases. This could be one way that too much saturated fat in the diet might contribute to disease.

By the end of our small intestine, the environment has become less acidic and more bacteria are thriving and multiplying. These include some that we know are good for us, such as the various *Lactobacillus* species that are found in good-quality yoghurts, kefir and cheeses, as well as other fermented foods. Yeasts also thrive here and, although when kept in balance with other bacteria they're not problematic, if the balance is disrupted (for example, after a dose of antibiotics) they can get out of control and cause problems such as candida. An allergic reaction to certain types of yeast is also thought to be involved in conditions such as Crohn's disease, coeliac disease and colitis. At the end of the small intestines our microbiota also create vitamin B_{12} for absorption into our system. This is just one of the very useful B-group vitamins that the microbiota synthesise for us.

Things get really interesting once the chyme (largely consisting by this stage of complex carbohydrates, or fibre, that couldn't be absorbed further up) moves into the large intestine (colon). This is where we see by far the largest number of bacteria living – estimates are about 1000 different species. These bacteria really like and need fibre, which comes from the different types of plant foods we eat. In fact, fibre is essential to our bacteria as they use it as a food source. This is a very important understanding, because we're all eating far less fibre than we used to and far less than we need to be eating for a healthy gut.

Currently the average daily intake of fibre for Australians is roughly 20 grams. The recommendations are for 25–30 grams per day, but people living traditional lifestyles in other countries can be consuming up to 100 grams of fibre per day, which is similar to human intakes in pre-agricultural times. We already know that fibre intake is strongly related to better health outcomes: people with diets higher in fibre are less likely to suffer from conditions such as hypertension, type 2 diabetes, dementia, depression and weight gain. This may well be because of the food this fibre provides for their gut bugs. Indeed, adding more fibre to our diet can shift our microbial profile from one linked to obesity to one associated with leanness.

When gut microbes ferment fibre from plant foods such as onions, garlic, artichokes, whole wheat, lentils and beans, and many other plant sources, they produce key molecules (metabolites) called short-chain fatty acids (SCFAs). These SCFAs, which include acetate, butyrate and propionate, have a multitude of actions in the body and brain. In fact, they interact with virtually every cell in the body. Particularly important may be the SCFA butyrate, which reduces inflammation and oxidative stress and maintains the health of the intestinal mucus lining. Fibre-rich plant foods feed the bugs that produce butyrate, giving us another pathway by which diet might influence our health. Unsurprisingly, people who eat a Mediterranean-style diet have much higher levels of bacterial diversity and SCFAs than those who don't. On the other hand, if we don't consume enough fibre then the bacteria can't do what they are supposed to do to run our body and brain. And it's not just the 'fermentable' fibre that is important. Recent research highlights the value of *non*-fermentable fibres such as those found in many types of wholegrain cereals, nuts and seeds and the skins of fruits and vegetables. Indeed, the main type of fibre – cellulose – that we get from fruits and vegetables is not fermented by our microbes to produce SCFAs. However, non-fermentable fibre seems to affect our gut in other ways. In a recent animal study focused on the processes behind multiple sclerosis (MS), non-fermentable dietary fibre altered the gut microbiota to increase *long*-chain fatty acids and prevented auto-immune disease developing. This points to the importance of diversity of types of fibre in our dietary intakes.

But why should we be thinking about these bugs, or what we should or shouldn't feed them, at all? Because we're increasingly certain that they play an important role not just in many aspects of our physical health and physiological processes, but also in our mental and brain health. And our diet seems to be the most important factor that influences the health (or otherwise) of our gut and its resident bugs.

The gut microbiota and mental and brain health

First, it's important to note that gut problems very commonly co-occur with depression. Our team has shown, using data from a large US study, that the most common physical symptoms accompanying depression are gut problems such as constipation, bloating and diarrhoea. Given the tight link between the gut and the brain, this isn't at all surprising to me. It may also be of relevance in ASD, where gut problems are very common.

The gut microbiota influences the brain via the vagus nerve using immune, hormone and neurotransmitter signalling. But this relationship goes both ways. Indeed, there's constant communication between the brain and the gut via what's known as the gut–brain axis. Most of the traffic (90 per cent) goes from the gut to the brain, but the brain also profoundly influences the gut. In particular, stress has a substantial impact on the gut and its resident bugs by changing gut motility. In simple terms, this means slowing down the transit of food through the gut. This makes sense, because our fight-or-flight (stress-response) system tells our body to move energy away from boring things like digestion to important things like running away from lions. But the changes in the gut environment have a big impact on which bugs live there and what they do, and in turn the health and functioning of the gut affects our immune system (among other things), giving us another way stress might affect our health.

Based on what we know so far, the gut microbiota play a key role in our immune functioning, metabolic processes (including glucose regulation and, importantly, body weight), stress-response system, brain health and brain plasticity, and gene expression. They also produce key neurotransmitters, such as dopamine, serotonin and gamma-aminobutyric acid (GABA). Indeed, more than 90 per cent of our body's serotonin is produced in our gut! While we don't think these neurotransmitters get through our blood–brain barrier, we do think they signal to the central nervous system via the gut–brain axis. We also know that the gut bacteria influence the metabolism of tryptophan, which affects serotonin production in the brain. Each of these processes or factors is also of real importance to our mental health, and how our brains develop and function throughout our life.

There's now compelling evidence from animal studies that the gut microbiota influence depressive and anxiety-like behaviours, and that changing the gut microbiota with specific probiotics or antibiotics, or even a poo transplant, can also influence these behaviours. In fact, recent studies have taken faeces from depressed people and transplanted them into animals, making the animals 'depressed' (indicated by depressive-like behaviours). This is quite amazing to me. Depression can actually be transmitted! Via a poo transplant! Swapping poo between different breeds of mice can also swap behavioural tendencies, making nervous mice calm and calm mice nervous. Researchers have shown that taking poo from a person with high blood pressure and putting it into a rodent can give the animal high blood pressure as well. You can even 'give' an animal obesity via a poo transplant from an obese human! All these studies tell us that the bacteria in our gut play an important role in our health.

Human studies using probiotics to improve mental health outcomes are starting to emerge as well. A very small study of 22 healthy men, conducted by my colleagues in Ireland, showed that giving a particular type of *Bifidobacteria* over a four-week period reduced anxiety and stress. They also saw improvements in cognitive function, particularly memory. A larger, randomised controlled trial in New Zealand has also been recently published. In this study of more than 400 women, those randomly assigned to receive a probiotic supplement containing *Lactobacillus* (*rhamnosus* HN001) over the course of their pregnancy and postpartum period had reduced levels of depression and anxiety compared to those receiving a placebo pill. We certainly need much more human research, but these intervention studies are hinting that we're on the right track with targeting the gut microbiota to alleviate mental health problems.

Gut microbes in infant brain and immune system development

Of particular relevance is the understanding that the gut microbiota in the first two to three years of life seems to be very important for brain development and the development of the immune system in infants. We know this from work in animal experiments, but increasingly the evidence from human studies is backing this up. We all have a particular microbial 'fingerprint', and it appears that this is pretty much established by the age of three. This means that what happens before that age can have a big impact on the health of the gut (and thus its host) throughout life.

We're not completely clear on how a mother's microbiome might influence the establishment of her child's microbiome, but children are certainly exposed (or 'seeded') with some of their mother's bugs during vaginal delivery. Babies born via caesarean section have a microbiome that more resembles the skin of their parents, and there's some evidence that this might predispose them to allergic diseases, autoimmune disorders and weight gain although we can't yet say for sure that this is because of microbiota. It may be because of the medical factors that led to the caesarean, or – and we'll discuss this further below – to the antibiotics that mum received as a result of the caesarean, which were then transmitted to the child.

Breastmilk seems to be another key way a baby receives bugs from their mum. In fact, as well as containing microbes, breastmilk contains complex sugars that feed the healthy *Lactobacillus* and special bugs called *Bifidobacteria*. These *Bifidobacteria* not only break down breastmilk in babies' guts but also educate their immune systems. This of course has implications for their long-term health, as it's in the early stages of a baby's life that their immune system is 'taught' to recognise which microbes might be pathogenic (that is, make them sick) or friendly. Without this training, the baby's immune system may end up attacking its own cells or friendly bacteria, which has implications for autoimmune disorders and a host of chronic health conditions (including depression) down the track. For example, children who are breastfed until they start to eat foods with gluten in them have only half the risk of developing coeliac disease, an autoimmune disorder. I don't think it's a coincidence that rates of autoimmune disorders, such as multiple sclerosis (MS), lupus, coeliac disease, inflammatory bowel diseases and type 1 diabetes, are rapidly increasing in the West. I believe it's at least partly to do with our impoverished guts, often exposed to antibiotics and poor diets right from the start of life, meaning that our immune systems are not properly trained.

A baby's gut and its resident microbiota are also very important for the development of the brain. Animals that are bred without any microbiota (called germ-free animals) have profound changes in their brains and behaviour. Indeed, they display behaviours that are similar to those seen in ASD, as well as a host of problems including reduced health of the blood–brain barrier, reduced brain plasticity, very different stress-response systems, and differences in their neurotransmitter systems. This is one of the key reasons we believe that the gut microbiota and diet in early life are so important to the development of a child's brain.

Many studies now tell us that pregnant animals fed unhealthy diets high in fats or low in fibre have offspring with a reduced diversity of bugs and increased gut inflammation. Most worrying is that research in animals has shown that after four generations of a low-fibre diet, many of the gut bacteria become extinct and can't be encouraged back again – even when fibre is reintroduced. I believe that this has very important implications for the future of human health, given that some bacterial species are unique and quite possibly essential to our functioning. Once they're extinct, this could spell real trouble. The context for this, of course, is the terrible diets of our children. Less than half a per cent of children and adolescents in Australia consume the recommended (minimum) of vegetables and legumes, which are primary sources of fibre in the diet. We may well be starving our bugs out of existence.

While delivery and breastfeeding both seem to be important in establishing a baby's gut microbiota, we think that it's what happens when a child makes the transition to solid food that's really important. And of course, this timing also coincides with babies beginning to crawl around on the ground and putting everything and anything into their mouths. There's a good reason for this – they're populating their guts. Children born into houses with pets and siblings have lower rates of allergic diseases, indicating better immune systems. This seems to be because they're getting exposed to more bugs and this helps 'train' their immune systems to be healthy. But children who are weaned onto foods with a good range (diversity) of plant foods, high in fibre and polyphenols, as well as a wide range of (whole) foods in general, are going to develop a far healthier and stronger gut microbiota than babies weaned onto a limited and/or unhealthy Western diet. Indeed, the gut microbiota of children in Africa – where they're exposed to soil, farm animals, and high-fibre, low-fat diets – have far greater diversity of bacteria and much higher levels of the SCFAs that the gut bugs produce when they ferment dietary fibre than do European children. They also have far lower rates of chronic diseases and allergies than children in the West.

Antibiotic use is another very important factor in establishing a child's gut microbiota – and its long-term health. While sometimes lifesaving, antibiotics, particularly when given very early in life (the first 12 months), can have a devastating impact on the gut microbial community. Sometimes this can be permanent. While antibiotics obviously must be used in serious health situations, they should be avoided wherever they're not strictly necessary. This goes for adults as well. Antibiotics given to mothers before delivery may have a detrimental effect on the microbiota of the infants and may be a reason we see these links between caesarean births and increased allergic diseases, autoimmune disorders and weight gain in children as they grow.

But it's not just the medical use of antibiotics that may be problematic. It's also thought that the antibiotics that have been used so extensively in the production of farm animals for human consumption (such as cattle and poultry) may have contributed to the obesity and allergic-disease epidemics we see in the West. In fact, the large majority of antibiotics are sold for use on farm animals rather than on people. And farmers often don't give the antibiotics just to treat sick animals, but rather 'just in case' to prevent diseases (and to fatten them up! Think about that for a moment). There aren't the same time limits on use in animals as there are in humans – in farm animals it's not uncommon for antibiotics to be used over an extended period of time, and this is contributing substantially to the emergence of antibiotic-resistant strains of bacteria. This is a really major, and scary, issue drawing a lot of attention in public health and policy discussions at the moment. Some people hope that our new knowledge of microbiota might allow us to find ways to mitigate the negative impact of antibiotics and even identify positive uses for these in enhancing gut health. But in the meantime, use antibiotics only when it's medically essential, which means only for serious bacterial conditions, and not for illnesses caused by viruses, which includes colds and flu. And if you do need to use them, take a course of probiotics immediately after.

Changing your gut microbes with diet

I mentioned that African children have healthier gut microbiota profiles than European children, and this is also the case in adults. In a fascinating study, researchers examined the gut microbiota and health of rural South Africans and African Americans. Obviously, their diets were very different, with the South Africans eating far more plant foods and less animal foods and fats than the African Americans, while the African Americans had diets high in processed foods, animal fats, added sugars and all the other things that go with Western diets. And their microbiota were also very different, with higher levels of microbial diversity and SCFAs in the rural South Africans compared to the African Americans. The levels of inflammation in the bowel were also much higher in the Americans. Such inflammation is linked to bowel cancer risk as well as other inflammatory bowel diseases. But what was really astonishing about this study was what happened when the researchers swapped the participants' diets for only two weeks. Levels of microbiota diversity and SCFAs went up in the African Americans and down in the South Africans, as did the markers of inflammation. *In two weeks.*

This tells us something very important that has now been backed up by other studies with humans: we can change the health of our gut very quickly by changing our diet. Another trial, which put ten healthy volunteers on either a 'plant-based' or 'animal-based' diet, showed a very rapid (five-day) change in the gut, with SCFAs going up in the plant-focused diet and down in the animal-foods diet. Gut profiles return to their baseline settings quickly after reverting to habitual diets, which also tells us that long-term dietary change is necessary to positively affect our gut and our health.

Diet and leaky gut

A key area of interest for researchers relates to the impact of different types of dietary fats on gut bacteria and gut health. High-fat diets in animal studies readily induce obesity, but also insulin resistance and – importantly – leaky gut. If you have an ongoing interest in diet and health, you may have heard this term before. I'll explain it briefly.

A healthy gut should have a nice, thick layer of mucus. This mucus layer helps to keep the contents of the gut where they're supposed to be – in the gut. When the lining of our gut is not covered by a healthy layer of mucus, however, the contents of the gut (bacteria, undigested food, toxins) can leak into the bloodstream. Our immune system mounts a defence response to this and it results in inflammation. It's even now thought that damage to the integrity of the gut lining, with the resulting inflammation, is another important driver of weight gain and obesity. It's also of real relevance to all the other aspects of our health that are affected by inflammation, including allergies, autoimmune disorders, asthma and inflammatory bowel disease, as well as depression and other mental health problems. Indeed, colleagues of mine examined this in a human study and saw evidence of leaky gut in people with clinical depression; they had higher levels of antibodies to bacteria in their blood than people without depression, suggesting that more of the bacteria were escaping the gut and getting into the bloodstream. This may also be a driver of the increased levels of inflammation that are commonly observed in people with a range of psychiatric diseases, including depression and psychosis.

Very importantly, when microbes are starved of fibre they can start to feed on this protective mucus lining of the gut, resulting in leaky gut. One study with mice sought to determine the possible impact of the diets many of us follow, where we might eat well one day but then have a day of unhealthy eating. They found that the mucus layer of these mice was half that of the mice kept on a high-fibre diet every day. This tells us that we need to keep it up! Of course, we've known for a long while that people who eat high-fibre diets lose weight and are better able to keep themselves in the healthy weight range. All of this provides very good incentives to increase our fibre intake.

But it's not just fibre we need to think about. Many animal studies tell us that high-fat diets can have a very detrimental impact on our gut lining. Understanding which fats are particularly problematic is one of the things we're working on at the moment. We know already that palm oil, which is high in saturated fat and very commonly used in making processed foods, seems to promote leaky gut and inflammation in animal experiments. A human study also shows that giving people palm oil for five weeks increased their LDL (the 'bad' type linked to heart disease) cholesterol. (As if that weren't enough, palm oil production is an important cause of deforestation and environmental destruction in places like Malaysia and Indonesia, including orangutan habitats, giving us another good reason to avoid processed foods.)

According to the evidence so far from animal studies, saturated fats promote dysbiosis (imbalance) of the gut microbiota and inflammation within the gut. As well as supporting the *Bilophila* bacteria, which as we have seen are pro-inflammatory, saturated fats seem to also promote bacteria that produce hydrogen sulfide gas. This in turns promotes damage to the gut lining. But it's not just saturated fats that are problematic for gut health: fats high in omega-6 fatty acids, such as corn oil (commonly used in processed foods), promote microbial dysbiosis and damage the gut lining. We've just done an animal study that compared different types of dietary fats on animal behaviour and have seen that soybean oil (also very commonly used in processed foods) seems to promote more anxiety-type behaviours than other sorts of oils, including butter, coconut oil and olive oil. On the other hand, it won't surprise you to hear that the omega-3 fatty acids, found in seafood and some nuts, as well as monounsaturated fats such as those found in olive oil and avocados, protect against microbial dysbiosis and help prevent insulin resistance and leaky gut. Interestingly, in one study the researchers noted that the detrimental impact on the gut microbiota that resulted from feeding animals butter was reversed by extra virgin olive oil but not refined olive oil. This likely relates to the importance of the non-lipid components of olive oil – the polyphenols. I'll now tell you something interesting about these polyphenols and body weight.

Diet, gut microbiota and body weight

It appears that our gut microbiota profoundly influence our tendency to gain weight. High-fibre diets are increasingly understood to be particularly important to losing weight or keeping it off because they provide the food that good bugs need to keep our metabolism ticking along healthily, as well as providing the 'bulk' in the diet that makes us feel full and displaces less healthy foods. But it also appears that gut bugs particularly appreciate polyphenols, which are valuable parts of fruit and vegetables, as well as of tea, coffee, red wine, olives and olive oil, and some herbs and spices. And polyphenols seem to play a role in reducing weight gain.

In two recent studies, researchers put rodents on three types of diet: their normal 'chow' diet, a high-fat diet, or a high-fat diet supplemented with added polyphenols. As expected, compared to the chow-fed group, the high-fat diet group put on weight and grew obese over the period of the study – this is what we would expect to see. The animals that were fed the high-fat diet with the added polyphenols, however, only put on about half as much weight as the high-fat diet group! Their trajectory of weight gain sat somewhere in the middle of the high-fat-only group and the chow group. What this is saying is that polyphenols in the diet may actually help us to avoid putting on weight, and this appears to happen by influencing our gut microbiota.

Intriguingly, the bugs themselves may play a part in food cravings, driving the consumption of foods that fuel bacterial fitness but not necessarily host health. In other words, bacteria that like fatty and sugary foods may send signals to the brain that prompt us to seek those sorts of foods. But increasing our microbial diversity by feeding ourselves and our families a wide range of whole foods may limit bacterial control over dietary cravings. This is another key piece of information that may help keep us within the healthy weight range.

Finally, I don't suppose I need to tell you that Western diets, with their added fats and sugars, are not good for your bugs. But there are a couple of other things about Western diets that I think you should know. First, artificial sugars, such as saccharin, aspartame and Splenda, have now been shown in animal studies to reduce beneficial bacteria such as *Bifidobacteria* and *Lactobacillus*, but also alter glucose regulation in a way that predisposes them to weight gain. This is at doses similar to what we'd be getting if we were regularly consuming diet soft drinks or other foods with added artificial sugars. In other words, even though they don't have their own calories, they might make us fat by changing our microbiota. There's a real irony in this, I think. Similarly, emulsifiers that are very commonly used in processed foods have now been shown to damage the gut. In effect, they act like detergent, stripping the very important mucus layer from our gut lining and promoting leaky gut. Finally, there's new evidence linking another common additive to processed foods – the sugar trehalose – to gut microbiota dysbiosis and the rise in a very nasty bowel infection caused by a bacterium called *Clostridium difficile*. So there are many good reasons to avoid processed foods, above and beyond their poor nutritional profile.

On the other hand, fermented foods such as kimchi, miso, soy sauce, tempeh, sauerkraut, non-processed cheese and yoghurt, all part of traditional diets, have important health benefits. They contain microorganisms themselves (probiotics), prebiotics (food for bugs) and metabolites, such as SCFAs, which are produced by bacteria during fermentation. These components may benefit gut microbiome composition and function, macronutrient breakdown and absorption, gut permeability and the gut immune system. Fermented foods also appear to have some anti-inflammatory and brain modulatory effects. We're very keen to soon start testing fermented foods as a strategy for improving gut and mental health in humans: stay tuned for those results.

All of this new information tells us that dietary manipulation, including eating more foods high in fibre, healthy fats, polyphenols and fermented foods, may result in positive changes in the activity of our microbiota and provide a feasible way of both preventing and treating depression and other disorders. Importantly, our diets go hand in hand with other health behaviours, such as exercise, sleep, smoking and alcohol consumption, that also influence microbial health. That said, so far diet seems to be the most important of these health behaviours.

Gut diversity: think of your gut as a rainforest

Scientists believe that having a higher level of bacterial diversity in the gut may be a marker of gut health; the more different types of bugs are there, the less chance there is that one species or another will dominate. It is also likely that the multiple rare species that a healthy gut harbours are ready to spring into action when we encounter an unusual food source; they are our mechanism of adaptation. Critically, having these rare species may help us to survive exposure to unusual pathogens that might otherwise kill us. Given the rise of antibiotic resistance, the chances of a new plague developing for which we have no treatment is growing. Having a diverse gut microbiota, with what Martin Blaser in his book *Missing Microbes* calls 'contingency species', might make the difference between survival or death. We need to think about our gut microbiota as an ecosystem or rainforest – diversity of life is a healthy sign of a complex system where all the elements work together. And the best way to encourage a diverse gut microbiota? Eat a diverse range of (whole) foods, particularly plant foods, and avoid the exposures that can negatively affect the ecosystem of our gut, such as antibiotics, processed foods, high levels of saturated fats, binge drinking and chronic stress.

There's a very interesting couple of microbiologist researchers in the United States, called the Sonnenburgs, who happen to be married to each other. They've done a lot of groundbreaking research into gut microbiota and health and have written a book about it, *The Good Gut*. They also have a young family and, based on their research (and their toddler's constipation), felt that it was important to increase their fibre intake and the bacterial diversity of their family's collective gut bugs. So they started to grow their own vegetables and other foods, even making their own sourdough breads. They also have pets and became a little less hung-up on 'cleanliness', reducing the use of common household disinfectants and the like. By doing this, they substantially increased the diversity of their gut microbiota. They focus on their diet in particular, ensuring a high intake of plant fibres from vegetables and fruits, wholegrains, beans and seeds – and that includes for their kids. As Justin said in a recent interview: 'You have to view what your kids are eating just like you view bedtime, going to school, buckling their seat belt. They may not want it, but it's what's best for them. You just tell them there's no option.'

Of course, when we all lived off the land or at least close to the land and our food sources, we were exposed to many different types of bacteria from our food. Not only does soil have enormous quantities of bacteria, but there are even bacteria *in* the vegetables themselves. But with large-scale agriculture, fruits and vegetables are now chlorinated, irradiated and 'sanitised' beyond recognition (from a microbial point of view).

AN IMPORTANT CAVEAT WITH GUT MICROBIOTA

It's important to bear in mind that the field of research focused on the gut microbiota is in its early stages and has not yet been able to comprehensively identify and describe the composition of a 'healthy' gut, nor the full functional capacity (what they do) of most types of bacteria. Overall microbiota composition and function can vary greatly between people, and different microbes can also have the same range of functions, making things even more complicated to investigate and understand. We're only at the beginning of the long task of unravelling how we interact with our bacteria partners, but the coming years should see huge strides in our knowledge.

Advances in technologies will continue to shed light on this rapidly developing field and, unlike the field of Nutritional Psychiatry, there are many, many researchers and research groups around the world currently focused on investigating this topic. In many ways, the gut microbiota is having as much of an impact on medical research as the discovery of very small particles did on the field of physics early last century. While new probiotic and dietary research tells us that the gut is likely to be a very important pathway by which diet, as well as other health behaviours and stress, influence mental and brain health, there's a clear need for more high-quality research. This is a key activity at our Food & Mood Centre.

Key facts

- The immune system and systemic inflammation are clearly related to mental disorders, including depression.
- Inflammation and its accompanying oxidative stress are often a result of mental illness, but also appear to be a causative factor.
- Diet quality is a key driver of immune function and inflammation.
- The size and function of the hippocampus (brain plasticity) appears to be influenced by diet, and healthier diets are linked to larger hippocampal size, while unhealthier diets are linked to smaller hippocampal size.
- Diet appears to regulate gene activity via a process called epigenetics, although this is a new field of research that requires more investigation.
- New evidence suggests that the gut microbiota drive immune function, metabolic processes and the health of the brain, and are a key determinant of human health.
- Research also suggests that gut microbiota influence mood and behaviour.
- Early-life gut microbiota seems to be critical for the development of the brain and immune system in infants. Particularly

important to establishing a healthy gut is breastfeeding and the quality of the diet that babies commence with solids feeding.

- Diet appears to be the most important factor influencing the health of the gut throughout life.
- Modification of the gut microbiome by dietary and related strategies may be useful in preventing and treating depression and other mental health problems.

9

If I improve my diet, will my mental health improve?

We now get to the crux of the matter and try to answer the $64 million question: I'm depressed – should I change my diet?

When I was approached to write this book, which was quite a while ago now, I said no – not yet, because I wanted to wait until I could give people information and guidance that was based on firm research evidence. So far, we've talked extensively about the evidence mainly from observational studies (where we don't change people's diets, but rather just record what they eat and measure their mental health) and from animal experiments. But, as we've discussed, there are limitations to what we can really know from these studies, as correlation doesn't necessarily equal causation and animals are not humans! Knowing that diet and mental health are related, or that dietary manipulation changes brain and behaviour in animals, is not the same as knowing that if you change diet, you change mental health in humans. Until the end of 2016, this was a question that had still not been answered.

But in early 2017 my team published the results of the first study to test the hypothesis that if you took people who had clinical depression and supported them to make improvements to their diet, their mood would improve. As we've discussed previously, such studies are challenging because getting people to improve their diet is not easy and we also can't 'blind' the participants to the nature of the study. We do, however, still need to conduct such studies to work out whether diet can be a useful strategy in clinical and real-world situations.

Happily, what we found was very encouraging, and it has had a big impact in the field of research and in the public domain. We've had news articles published all over the world, including in the *Wall Street Journal*, *The Atlantic*, BBC Science, NBC and many others, and it's still reverberating. We didn't expect that it would have such an impact, but I think it was simply the right study at the right time. It's been many decades since we've had any truly new treatments for depression, and the ones we do have only help some people. The idea that changing diet might help improve our mental health, as well as our physical health, really appeals to people. Apart from anything else, it gives them the power to take action for themselves, and this seems to be something they really respond to. I'm going to give you some detail here about what we did and how we did it, but *why* we did it should be obvious by now.

The SMILES study

Our Supporting the Modification of Lifestyles in Lowered Emotional States (SMILES) study was the logical next step after all the research work we'd done using observational methods. But it took quite a lot of thinking and planning to develop a protocol that we could use to test the hypothesis in a way that was scientifically rigorous, given the issues related to dietary intervention studies. I consulted many people to try to find the best way forward, and was eventually successful in obtaining some funding from our National Health and Medical Research Council to run the study.

The aim of the study was to see whether helping people to improve their diets would have a meaningful impact on their depressive symptoms. To do this, we aimed to recruit nearly 180 people – men and women – with clinical depression (major depressive disorder), and to randomly assign them to either a dietary support group or a social support group. Social support in this type of study consists of meeting with a research assistant to discuss neutral topics of interest, such as a person's hobbies and passions, but doesn't involve counselling. We know that social support (simply speaking, having someone to take an interest in us and with whom we can spend some time talking) is helpful for people with depression. But the other reason we chose this as a comparison group was because we needed to control for the non-specific effects of seeing a dietitian.

If someone sees a health practitioner, such as a dietitian, of course they don't just receive dietary support. They also receive social support, as a good-quality clinician takes an interest in their clients, listens to them, chats with them, and often offers them feedback and support over and above any discussion of diet. So we needed to make sure that the people in the non-dietary group were receiving some sort of support that was of an equivalent nature, while not involving any dietary education or counselling.

The people assigned to the dietary support group received individual guidance from a clinical dietitian to make improvements to their diets. I had as one of my key collaborators Professor Catherine Itsiopoulos, who is a world expert on the Mediterranean diet. She helped our mutual PhD student at the time, Rachelle Opie, to develop a diet that we felt would tick all the boxes for mental health, based on our previous research. This diet was based on a traditional Mediterranean diet, with a focus on vegetables, fruit, legumes, nuts, whole grains, fish and olive oil. But in contrast to a traditional Mediterranean diet, it also included recommendations to consume small serves of unprocessed red meat three to four times per week. This was because of our previous finding regarding red meat and depressive and anxiety disorders and symptoms in women (more about this in Chapter 11).

Both groups saw someone – either a research assistant or a dietitian – weekly, then fortnightly, over a three-month period for a total of seven sessions. Participants could continue on their current treatment, whether antidepressants, counselling or both, so this was what was known as an 'adjunctive' trial – in other words, the intervention was in addition to – not instead of – other forms of treatment. (This is important to emphasise: I would never suggest that a healthy diet should replace other forms of treatment. I have benefitted greatly from a very low-dose antidepressant at times. Given my history of clinical depression and anxiety and my high genetic load, this has been very helpful in combination with a healthy diet, exercise and sleep.)

I don't mind telling you that this was a very difficult study to do. The first and main reason was that we had real difficulties recruiting people to the study. There were a few reasons for this, I think. First, people with major depression often suffer from profound fatigue and a lack of energy and interest that makes leaving the house and attending regular appointments very challenging for them. Secondly – as is the case with many of these sorts of randomised, controlled trials – many potential participants were put off by the fact that they had a 50–50 chance of receiving social support rather than dietary support. I think there might also have been a general feeling from people that dietary change wasn't going to do much for the depression so why bother. Or that changing diet was just going to be too difficult. Finally, and I think this is a key factor, we didn't have support of doctors and psychiatrists referring their patients to the study.

This is a common problem in any trials in psychiatry or medicine, but in our case I think that the level of scepticism from medical practitioners about the usefulness of our approach meant there was little support from the medical fraternity. As a result, we were only able to recruit, after three long, hard years of trying, 67 people to the study. Having said that, the people who did come into the study were happy with their experience and – importantly – the ones in the dietary group were able to make the positive changes they needed to their diets with the support of the dietitians.

It's important to understand that to get into the study, people had to have a poor diet to start with. As you might imagine, with less than 10 per cent of the general population eating according to the dietary guidelines, then with the added pressures of depression, this was a very easy criterion for most people to fulfil and we excluded only a handful of potential participants because their diets were too healthy! The job of the dietitians was to help participants to reduce their intake of 'extras' foods – crisps, sweets, desserts, cakes, doughnuts and pastries, fast foods and packaged foods – and to increase their intake of whole foods. The participants were gently supported to replace their white breads with wholegrain and sourdough breads; their sweet, processed cereals with unsweetened muesli and oats; their pizzas with vegetable stir-fries; their ham, sausages and bacon with fish and small amounts of lean red meats; their sweets with fresh fruit; and to include beans, legumes and nuts in their meals and snacks, and use olive oil for all their cooking and salads. They were given a hamper at the start of the study with a few examples and 'tasters' of the sorts of foods we wanted them to eat. Very importantly, the dietitians supported the individual participants to set realistic goals and took a non-judgemental and personalised approach. You can read more details of the SMILES study diet – which Rachelle named the ModiMed diet – in Chapter 12 and the Appendix, but it's important to note that it wasn't a diet that had to be rigorously adhered to, with measuring, weighing and recording of food. Rather, it was designed to be inexpensive and achievable, and to give people the tools they needed to make long-term, positive changes to their diet.

To be honest, I don't think any of us really expected to find a difference in the participants' depressive symptoms at the end of the 12-week study, particularly given that we had such a small sample size. Having so few people in the study meant that there needed to be a very big difference in the average depression scores between the groups at the end of the study for us to be able to detect it statistically. Maybe, deep down, I was as sceptical as anyone else about the ability of dietary change to affect such a serious disorder as major depression. You can imagine my surprise and excitement when the statistician did the analyses and we saw that there was – in fact – a very big difference between the two groups. While the average depression scores improved in both groups, which is what you'll almost always see with a trial in depression, the scores improved far more in the dietary support group, with roughly a third of the people in that group going into remission (that means, no longer classified as depressed) compared to 8 per cent in the social support group. We had what is known as a large 'effect size', meaning that it was a pretty big difference.

We checked, and this change and improvement wasn't due to people changing their exercise habits or losing weight. This is important, because – as we previously discussed – the association between diet quality and mental health seems to exist quite independently of weight. Our diet did not have a weight-loss focus, and participants were encouraged to eat according to their hunger. Given that, we didn't expect people's weight to change – and it didn't. In our study, the average BMI was roughly 30, meaning that most people in the study were overweight or obese, and that didn't change during the trial. What did change, however, was people's depression and – possibly most importantly of all – it changed in line with dietary change. Simply speaking, this meant that the more people improved their diets, the more their depression improved. And people seemed to really like this approach. This is what one of our participants said:

> Having had four to five cycles of major depression I found neither talk therapy nor medication of help. In fact, these methods, in my particular case, made the experience worse.
>
> However, the SMILES trial did help – so much so that I follow it today, four years later. The program was to me a last resort. With its success, I am forever grateful.
>
> I believe it is partly the food, and partly the focus provided (positive yet accountable) that is of benefit. Therefore, I would wholeheartedly support the recommendation of including a clinical nutritionist within the allied health team for those suffering major depression.

Eating healthily needn't be expensive

Now I'm going to tell you something else that is nearly as important as the findings of the study itself, and that's the results of the economic evaluation of the study. This is termed the 'cost-effectiveness', and these evaluations were done by health economists who were on the study team. They considered 'societal costs', which included the cost of delivering the interventions (i.e. the wages of the research assistants and the dietitians), as well as the cost of food, and travel costs to and from the study centre. Health-sector costs took into account the costs of medications and medical services, and absenteeism and presenteesim from paid and unpaid duties, such as paid work and domestic duties.

Again, we were all surprised by the results. Compared with the social support group, average health-sector costs for the dietary support group were $856 lower, and average societal costs were $2591 lower. These differences were driven by lower costs arising from fewer allied and other health professional visits and lower costs of unpaid productivity. In other words, people in the dietary support group saw health practitioners less often during the study and lost less time from their unpaid roles (that is, domestic duties, volunteering, child care and the like). Accordingly, the conclusion was that our approach was 'likely cost-effective as an adjunctive treatment for depression from both health sector and societal perspectives'.

Now this is very important for a key reason – if you want to change policies, you need to change the mind of politicians. And to do this, you need to show them that they can save money by adopting your recommendations. Our findings suggested that people being treated for depression using a dietary approach experienced a benefit to their overall health, evidenced by fewer trips to health professionals and less time when they couldn't undertake their daily duties. And this points to another critical point: having depression increases the risk of heart disease, obesity and metabolic syndrome, while these conditions – in turn – increase the risk of depression. In other words, depression and common, chronic health conditions are very often 'comorbid' (meaning that they co-occur) but are also mutually reinforcing. If we can successfully take a dietary approach to treating depression, it's very likely to have a benefit for all the other chronic diseases that we know are so common and that present such an enormous challenge to society and the public purse.

There's one final point I'd like to make about our SMILES study, as it's one we're often asked about. There's a common belief that to eat a healthy diet, you have to spend more money than that needed to eat an unhealthy diet. I'm not saying that that's not the case in countries such as the United States, where their food system is fundamentally changed (broken, I would say) and where 'food deserts and swamps' are common (these are areas where fast-food outlets are plentiful, with their extremely cheap, upsized burgers, fries and soda, and where fresh food is hard to get and more expensive). In many other countries, however – and certainly in Australia – whole foods are plentiful unless you're in a very remote area, and it's a matter of making sensible choices with your shopping.

Dr Rachelle Opie, during the SMILES study, undertook an extremely detailed cost analysis of the diets people were eating when they started the study, with higher intakes of 'extras' foods, and compared it to the costs of the diet we were recommending. What she found goes against this belief that a healthy diet needs to be more expensive than an unhealthy one. She found, in fact, that the average per-person cost of the diet she'd designed for the SMILES participants was *cheaper* than the diets participants were on when they started the study. At the start of the study, trial participants spent an average of $138 per week on food and beverages for personal consumption, while the average food and beverage costs per person per week for our recommended diet was only $112.

There are a few caveats with this. If you were to decide to change your diet and head off to the shops to overhaul your pantry, you could really do a lot of damage to your wallet if you made the wrong choices. For example, if you decided to go all organic, or to buy fresh berries, fish and the finest cuts of meat, or lots of prepackaged 'healthy' meals, you'd soon find a big hole in your pocket. But if you were canny and chose tinned fish, tinned or dried legumes (lentils, chickpeas, beans), and fresh or even frozen vegetables (nutritionally just as good), and you used foods that were local and in season rather than imported and out of season, then your money would go a lot further. And this is what the dietitians recommended on the SMILES trial. We'll give you the details and suggestions from the trial in Chapter 12 and the Appendix.

How the SMILES study changed lives

But now I'd like to leave you with another bit of feedback from another of the SMILES participants – let's call him Aaron. This sort of message is what researchers like me live for – knowing that we've been able to help someone is what keeps us going every day.

By 2012 I had grown to appreciate how poor my mental health had become. I was desperate for anything that might help. So I signed up for every promising research study I could find. SMILES was the most involved, longest running and – as far as I remember – the most helpful of them.

The impact of the trial to my lifestyle cannot be understated. My diet radically shifted and I have maintained those key changes. I was able to adapt the dietary intervention around my rather fussy eating pattern and on-and-off-again vegetarianism – in fact, the intervention changed my attitude to food in some ways. I wasn't a perfect subject by any means – I experimented with the fish and red meat but couldn't stomach it – but encouragement and access to high-quality ingredients and the practice of cooking boosted my sense of effectiveness and self-worth in any case.

Long after the trial, when my eating habits would lapse, I'd notice my mental health also wavered. Practically speaking, I felt much better after I had made the changes. I felt better about the way I was living, the choices I had made, and the food itself gave me a higher, more stable and cleaner mood than before. I began to identify as someone who cared about their health and well-being, and this cascaded into other changes. I improved my sleep hygiene, started exercising and stressed less about university.

Funnily enough, I went from a student who had failed six out of my eight subjects to date, under review by the academic committee, to a high-performing student with no further fails, who scraped into a postgraduate epidemiology degree outside my original area of interest, geology, by taking some agricultural science units. My interest in epidemiology was sparked by my eye-witness experience of how medical research can turn some-one's life around.

Today, I work on health and medical research policy for the Department of Health. To this day, every flick of my wrist for a splash of extra virgin olive oil or a handful of brain-shaped walnuts, foods I started eating during the trial, reminds me that food and mood go hand in hand.

Here's another message from one of the SMILES trial participants, who did some media interviews for us after she finished the trial. It's been several years since she took part, and it was fascinating to see how she's going now and so gratifying to know that we were able to help her.

The first thing I can say is that the SMILES trial saved my life. When I found the advertisement on the internet I was lying in bed in the middle of the day crying and seriously contemplating ending my life. My body hurt, my mind hurt, and I was exhausted. I was drinking a bottle of wine every night and smoking half a packet of cigarettes a day. I was on 300 mg of Zoloft a day, with my psychiatrist saying that I would have to be on the drug for the rest of my life. My marriage was on the rocks and the only thing that kept me going was my two daughters. I did not know what else to do but end it all. But obviously that was no good for anyone.

In the back of my mind I could hear someone saying, 'There is always new treatment for different illnesses.' So I googled research treatment for depression and I came across the information to your trial. I applied and thought I would never hear back but the next day, Sarah [one of our wonderful research assistants] emailed me and got the ball rolling. I jumped at the chance and thought it was worth a try since nothing else had worked.

Within two weeks of meeting Sarah and Rachelle, who advised me that I would be participating on the nutritional side of things, I started feeling like there was hope. I have always been a big believer in eating well; however, when suffering from depression, it was very difficult to feed the family, let alone myself.

After my first session with Rachelle and learning what I would and should be eating, I felt in control and empowered to try to get out of this black hole that I was drowning in.

As the trial went on, I ate more and more good food. I was never a processed-food junkie, but my biggest problem was that I didn't eat enough and I lived on coffee, wine and cigarettes. The coffee and the cigarettes stayed for a while, but the wine started to disappear. I didn't feel the need for it and I started craving better food. I finally had an appetite again.

By the end of the trial I was well on my way to feeling good again. I was motivated to learn more about nutrition and I thought I could use my experience to help others, so I began my Diploma of Health Science (nutritional medicine).

I studied for a year of a two-year course, but then things started to fall down again. I was getting out of the habit of eating my good healthy food as the stress of studying and being a mother and housewife was becoming too much. I quit the course and started to fall into the black hole again. I started feeling less motivated and scared that I was going backwards.

I was very fortunate to get in contact with an old school friend who had suffered a similar illness. We reconnected, and he gave me the motivation to start to eat better again. We would chat about the issues we had and how the food affected our moods. It was once again a lifesaver, and I value his friendship 15 months later.

Now on the right track again, armed with the information that I received on the trial, I soldiered on. Taking note of how I felt after I ate certain things, I started researching more and more, especially whole and raw foods. I started exercising by walking 4–5 kilometres a couple of times a week. I realised this was something I really enjoyed doing. I was always interested in hiking, and after reconnecting with my school buddy and finding out that he was also into hiking, I found someone with a common interest.

I joined a couple of 'meet-up' groups and found a great group and started regular hikes with them. This gave me the motivation to continue eating well, and I started to give up the cigarettes. You just can't get up those hills with a lungful of nicotine and poison.

Then, in June 2017, my husband and I decided we would move our family back to our hometown of Brisbane. We are both originally from Brisbane and moved to Melbourne for his work. Now, 14 years later, we had our two daughters and I thought it was time to go home. So that journey began. We had to convince our daughters and consider my parents' (who lived with us) needs for the big move. After much discussion, we decided to put the house on the market and take the leap. This was extremely stressful, leaving routine, friends and a familiar community. There were a lot of emotions going through my mind about moving back to a city that held so many uneasy memories for me. I wasn't sure if it was the best thing.

I continued to fuel my body with nutrient-dense food and got out hiking as much as possible. I had even joined a gym for the cold and rainy Melbourne winter days, as I was becoming more aware of how I felt after I had walked 15–20 kilometre hikes. Exercise has played a huge part in my recovery, and I believe that this has given me the strength to believe in myself and the courage to face a few demons that I had buried long ago.

So, on 8 January this year we arrived in Brisbane to start our new life. I have continued to hike and eat well and I am now four weeks out of completing my first endurance hiking event. On 22 June I will be walking 100 kilometres for Oxfam. Without good food I would never have been able to train like I have. I am very mindful of how my mind works and how my body feels if I have been eating well and exercising compared to not eating well and lying around.

There are certainly things in my life that aren't perfect, but hey, who lives a perfect life? Now I am stronger, I am able to cope with stresses that life will throw at me. Depression attacks these coping skills, and that is what pushes you into the black hole.

If I am feeling yuk and I just don't care what I eat or not eat, and I know that if I don't have something good I will get so much worse, I have my survival food. I always have fresh vegies in the fridge and some soup in the freezer. Heating this up is a nice comfort and nutritious boost, and I give myself time to rest. My husband knows that it is what I need when I just can't do it that day. This is my mental health first aid. I would recommend everyone has some sort of healthy comfort go-to food for 'those days' instead of reaching for the takeaway.

I have lost 5 kilograms and gone down a dress size. I still drink my coffee, but I stick to decaf after midday. I have the odd glass of wine with friends but two glasses and that is enough. I am very proud to say that the cigarettes have certainly not followed me to Brisbane. I have joined a gym with two strength classes a week, a night-training hike and a boxing class to punch out those frustrations.

I have also been very fortunate to be able to train with a school buddy who lives in Brisbane. I train with him once or twice a week as he has a team for Oxfam. My team consists of two girls from interstate and yet another school friend that I have not seen for many years and was always someone I found quite intimidating at school, but I now have the strength and confidence to believe in myself and not let the old feelings pull me into the hole that I was once in.

In the past 12 months I have also been able to reduce my medication from 300 mg to 150 mg all while moving. I am so proud of myself and I thank you all every moment for helping me and saving my life.

I thoroughly enjoyed doing the media interviews, as I think that getting the message out there and having the conversation about this horrible and debilitating issue is so important. I remember having mums from my daughters' school just hug me and saying thank you for inspiring them to look at their lives and their food. I hope that I have been able to empower others to educate themselves on the foods that will save them. Your trial has been the best thing that has happened to me and I thank you!

Like I said, it's stories like these that get me out of bed every day.

The HELFIMED study

I now want to discuss a second study that has just been published by colleagues of mine in South Australia; it backs up and extends our findings beautifully.

In the HELFIMED study, adults with depression were randomly assigned to a dietary group or a social group, similar to our SMILES study design. Instead of individual counselling with a clinical dietitian, however, those in the HELFIMED dietary group received group cooking workshops, teaching them the basics of a Mediterranean-style diet, plus fortnightly food hampers and fish oil supplements.

In the first visit, those in the dietary group were given an interactive nutrition education session led by a clinical dietitian and a nutritionist. For their subsequent fortnightly visits, they took part in cooking workshops where recipes focused on simple, healthy, affordable, tasty meals using Mediterranean dietary principles. Following the cooking workshop, the dietary participants were given food hampers that provided ingredients for the recipe that had been cooked, along with extra virgin olive oil, vegetables, fruit, tinned legumes, tinned tomatoes, tinned tuna and mixed nuts (almonds, walnuts and hazelnuts – the same nuts as in the PREDIMED study). They were also provided with recipes, cooking videos and other resources.

In common with our study, the design of HELFIMED controlled for the social interaction component of the cooking workshops by having an active 'social' comparison group. Participants in this group met fortnightly to participate in a range of social activities, such as playing games and book-club activities. Many participants in both groups formed friendships as a result of the shared activities, which is of course beneficial for depression. The main study ran for three months and involved a larger sample size than ours (more than 150 participants). As in SMILES, the participants in HELFIMED could continue with their current treatments, whether medications, counselling or both.

Happily, the HELFIMED workshops were highly successful at helping people to change their diets; those in the dietary group increased the amount and diversity of vegetables they ate, and also increased their intake of fruit, wholegrain foods, nuts and legumes, and reduced their unhealthy snacks. And both groups improved their depression; this makes sense, as group-based peer support has been shown to be as effective for treating depression as psychotherapy. In common with our study, however, the symptoms of those in the dietary group improved substantially more than those in the social group. In fact, it was striking just how similar the findings were from this trial to ours – we could virtually overlay the graphs on each other.

And, again, the degree of dietary improvement was linked to the improvement in symptoms – the more people improved their diet quality, the more they reported their depression and anxiety reduced, and quality of life increased. Another great outcome of this study was the finding that the benefits to people's diet quality, mental health and quality of life were sustained when they were assessed three months after the end of the study. This suggests that learning basic cooking skills and the hands-on learning of healthy recipes supported participants to make sustainable, long-term improvements to their dietary habits, and that this continued to contribute to better mental (and probably physical) functioning.

Because we and the HELFIMED team couldn't blind people to the nature of the intervention, and the associated issue of 'expectation bias' (people believing that dietary change was going to improve their symptoms resulting in a placebo response), we can't say absolutely that it was the dietary changes that effected the improvements in depression in these studies. But if we consider the weight of the observational and animal evidence, as well as the biological plausibility of diet as a factor affecting mental and brain health, I think there's pretty good evidence now that we can, indeed, treat at least some cases of depression using a dietary approach. Certainly, there was a strong relationship between the extent of dietary improvement and the degree of improvement in depression in both studies, which supports a direct effect.

Can we prevent mental disorders with dietary change?

Finally, I'm going to tell you about an intervention study that – along with all the observational evidence – suggests we may also be able to prevent depression happening in the first place.

In previous chapters, I've spoken about the large PREDIMED study, which showed that older people at higher risk of cardiac events could lower their risk of these, and of cognitive decline, by adopting a Mediterranean diet. Although the study wasn't set up to do this, my colleagues in Spain analysed the data from the PREDIMED study to see if there was any impact of a Mediterranean diet on depression risk. Because most new 'cases' of depression manifest early in life, to test this hypothesis properly the study would have needed to have many more study participants – maybe as many as 30,000 or more. After the researchers had excluded those who had been in the study for less than three years or, importantly, had reported previous depression, there were only about 4000 people to study. Still, they thought that it was worth investigating and what they found was interesting.

Even though they really didn't have a large enough sample size (which limited what is known as their 'statistical power') they saw that at the end of the study, people who had changed to a Mediterranean diet with extra nuts tended to be less likely to have developed a new depressive illness compared to those who were on the low-fat control diet. And in the people with type 2 diabetes, who comprised approximately half the sample, that finding was statistically significant. This suggests that a Mediterranean diet (we don't know whether or not the raw nuts are particularly important) might be able to prevent the development of depression in older adults, particularly those with diabetes. This is consistent with another observational study we conducted with data from a large study in the United States; we saw that people with a healthy dietary pattern were less likely to have depression, and that the relationship between healthy diet and less depression was particularly strong in those with type 2 diabetes. It may be that in those who already have dysregulated glucose metabolism (in other words, type 2 diabetes), a healthy diet is even more important in reducing the risk of depressive illness.

Key facts

- Whether in one-on-one or group-based settings, giving people with depression guidance, support, feedback and information can help them improve the quality of their diet.
- Such dietary improvements appear to have large benefits for their depressive symptoms.
- A healthy diet doesn't need to be expensive; in fact, it can be cheaper than an unhealthy diet.

- Taking a dietary approach to treating depression appears to be highly cost-effective.
- The evidence from the PREDIMED study suggests that making positive changes to our diet might help prevent us developing depression as we age.

10

How can we improve things?

It seems clear to me that taking a holistic approach to treating mental health problems makes every kind of sense. First, even without knowing that improving diet can improve mental health in sufferers, the fact that people with mental health problems are at increased risk of heart disease, diabetes, obesity and metabolic syndrome suggests that targeting lifestyle behaviours is a particularly important first step in treating people with mental health problems. Happily, at least in Australia, we're starting to make some moves towards this approach.

How can we change clinical practices?

The updated clinical guidelines for the treatment of mood disorders (depressive and bipolar disorders) in Australia, published by the Royal Australian and New Zealand College of Psychiatrists in 2015, recommend targeting diet, exercise, smoking and sleep as the first steps for clinicians when they have a patient with a mood disorder, before they move onto considering other forms of treatment. That doesn't mean that this is routinely done in clinical practice though – putting out guidelines doesn't necessarily translate into changes in the way medical practitioners treat their patients. This is why we needed to do studies that specifically evaluate the usefulness of changing diet for people with depression, which is of course the most common of the mental health problems. Now that we have this new evidence, there's even more reason for medical practitioners to start treating the whole person, and not just bits of their brain.

We need to educate our health practitioners

We really need to beef up the education on nutrition that is given to medical practitioners. Most doctors and psychiatrists would have received very little information on nutrition as part of their training, and I know, from talking to many of them, that they're often unsure what to recommend to patients or where to find out about diet. Surveys in the United States tell us that three-quarters of junior doctors feel inadequately trained for counselling their patients about diet and exercise. The UK surveys tell us the same thing. One of the tasks we're currently undertaking at the Food & Mood Centre is to develop graduate training courses for health professionals, along with a textbook, as well as to contribute new content to the training given in our own university's health degrees. This is a good start, and these approaches will – I hope – become more widespread in the near future.

Health practitioners need to change their recommendations

I don't believe that making dietary recommendations to patients needs to be complicated. Two of my US psychiatry colleagues,

Dr Drew Ramsey from Columbia University and Dr Emily Deans in Boston, have been vocal and high-profile proponents of a new approach to psychiatry where nutrition is front and centre of the treatment regime. They recommend simply starting the conversation with a patient: 'Can you tell me about what you eat? What about for breakfast? Lunch? Dinner? Snacks and favourite foods? Aversions, allergies?' Then assessing the patient's openness and motivation to change and using motivational interview techniques to gently discuss options for replacing low-yield foods (i.e. foods low in nutrition and high in refined carbohydrates, added sugars, fats and salt) with high-yield foods, such as seafood, vegetables, grass-fed meats, whole grains, nuts and legumes. This should go along with strong recommendations to get moving, as even small increases in physical activity (it doesn't even need to be aerobic – it can be weight/resistance training or simply walking) can improve depression. I think that, based on all the evidence, diet and exercise should be an actual prescription from the doctor or psychiatrists, written down just as a prescription for a medication might be.

We need to change foods in hospitals

The menus and food environment in our hospitals and psychiatric inpatient units also need to be evaluated and substantially changed, in order to support people's recovery and to send the right messages. Currently, inpatients will have access to vending machines full of snack foods and their meal options are often high in refined carbohydrates, added sugar and salt, and very low in fibre and healthy fats. Here's one example: a facility in my city for young people with serious mental health problems currently gives its inpatients sweet muffins for snacks. This sends all the wrong messages and really won't help their recovery.

The young people also now use Uber to order in fast food, delivered directly to them in the hospital! It's a very difficult and tricky thing to change, but I know that many of my psychiatrist colleagues are working on auditing the current situation and beginning the long and fraught process of improvement.

It's challenging to overhaul a hospital kitchen's practices – I'm told there's often much resistance from the doctors and nurses, whose diets and lifestyle behaviours can be as bad as those of the patients', as well as from the hospital boards, which are concerned with costs. There is, however, plenty of scope to implement easier options in the short term: day programs and group-based cooking workshops are a great starting point. The HELFIMED study showed how popular and effective these can be. The researchers also noted that as participants cooked and ate together, they gradually became more socially engaged and built friendships. This is an obvious added bonus of cooking classes, and the Mediterranean diet, with its emphasis on the communal nature of eating, is a great template to follow.

We need clinical dietitians

Finally, I'd like to make a point about clinical dietitians. Before we started our SMILES study we did a review of the literature to assess what other studies existed where an approach to changing lifestyle had been attempted and mental health had been measured as an outcome. Although no studies had tried to implement a dietary program specifically for clinical depression, there were studies in people with other medical conditions, about half of which had shown a benefit to mental health symptoms. The key factor that seemed to determine whether or not the program was successful was the use of a clinical dietitian to deliver the intervention, rather than a research assistant or non-clinical nutritionist.

This makes sense, as a big part of a clinical dietitian's training deals with not 'what' but 'how'. In other words, the ability to assess where someone is at in terms of their readiness to make changes, then to use personalised strategies and motivational interviewing techniques to help them gradually make the necessary changes to their diet.

To my mind, one of the easiest things governments could do to translate this new evidence into meaningful benefits to the community would be to ensure access to clinical dietitians as part of primary care and mental health care teams. In Australia, where we have a universal healthcare system, people with depression who go to see their doctor (and this is the first stop for most people with depression) can see a psychologist for free for a certain number of sessions every year, as well as get a prescription for antidepressants. But if they go to a doctor with chronic medical conditions, such as type 2 diabetes, they can have several sessions with a dietitian for free. My thinking is that making dietitians available to people with depression – in other words, more commonly recognising depression as a chronic medical condition, with many of the same underlying biological and lifestyle determinants as heart disease, type 2 diabetes, obesity and the like – would be an obvious and relatively straightforward change that could be enacted quite quickly.

Similarly, ensuring that people with serious mental illnesses such as schizophrenia also have dietitians, as well as exercise physiologists, as part of the standard treatment team is a no-brainer as far as I'm concerned. You might remember the important work I mentioned earlier from colleagues of mine in Sydney who are pioneering lifestyle programs for people with serious mental illnesses (SMIs) such as psychotic disorders. Why is it important to support people with SMIs to adopt healthy lifestyle habits?

Because of some shocking statistics: in Australia, people with schizophrenia die, on average, 20 years earlier than people in the general population. Obesity affects 40–60 per cent of people with schizophrenia, and the large majority of people with SMIs experience substantial weight gain once they commence treatment with antipsychotic medications (which affect glucose regulation). Depending on how it's measured, roughly 20 per cent of Australians have metabolic syndrome, yet that figure is closer to 70 per cent in those with schizophrenia. Similarly, smoking rates in people with SMIs in Australia are four to five times higher than in the general population, and people with SMIs are far less likely to quit smoking. All of these figures translate to a significantly increased risk of early death from a whole range of diseases, such as type 2 diabetes, heart disease, pneumonia, influenza and circulatory diseases, in those with SMIs. So lifestyle programs that help people with these disorders to improve their diet, exercise and smoking habits, and thus mitigate the terrible impact of these illnesses on their long-term health and quality of life, are critical for reasons of equity as well as cost-effectiveness.

We need to advise pregnant women

Another strategy I think is well overdue is placing more emphasis on the importance of nutrition for women in the pre- and perinatal period. We know that – in common with the rest of the population – only about 10 per cent of pregnant women in Australia adhere to the national guidelines for healthy eating. Even worse, there's evidence that women's diets often get worse during pregnancy! Part of the reason for this is the warnings that pregnant women are given about what to avoid (raw fish, soft cheeses, unwashed salads) to reduce their risk of pathogens such as listeria and toxoplasmosis that are particularly dangerous during pregnancy.

Unfortunately, this often results in women unnecessarily restricting their diets and avoiding a range of healthy foods, such as fish and salads, in favour of processed 'safe' foods. Given what we know about the importance of good nutrition for both mothers' and children's emotional health, plus the detrimental impact of maternal obesity, high blood glucose and metabolic syndrome on child neurodevelopment, public health messages and clinical programs for women during pregnancy, focusing on nutrition, should be developed and evaluated. Of course, ideally this needs to happen way before pregnancy, and a range of important strategies and changes need to be implemented to help children, adolescents and then young adults – who go onto become parents – to avoid becoming metabolically unhealthy in the first place. For more about this, see below.

While I don't believe it will happen overnight, the new push to recognise food as essential to health, including mental health, means that there's growing grassroots support for these changes. Once a ground-swell starts to happen, things tend to take on their own momentum, so I feel optimistic about the future of clinical practice in psychiatry.

What can policymakers do?

I took leave in Bali to complete this book, and my experience provides a very good illustration of the massive scale of the problems we face.

When my husband and I first arrived, we visited a large supermarket to stock up on groceries for our stay. I was astonished and quite devastated, but maybe not surprised, to see that roughly half the supermarket was given over to packaged foods of the worst kind. There were aisles and aisles of packaged noodles, full of highly refined wheat, fats and salt and virtually no nutrition; endless packs of refined seed oils (which are full of the wrong sorts of fatty acids); rows and rows of sugar-sweetened drinks in bottles and cartons; and a seemingly endless supply of highly processed snack foods, including cakes, biscuits, fried snacks and sweets. Only a small section of the supermarket had fresh food for sale. All around us in Indonesia is the evidence of what is called the 'nutritional transition'; many people, predominantly children and young people, are clearly overweight and obese, while the older Balinese, after a lifetime of a traditional Balinese diet of fresh chicken or pork, rice, vegetables and fruit, are still lean.

This is the transition underway across the globe as we speak, and it's heartbreaking. This is the reality behind those statistics discussed at the start of the book: unhealthy diet as the leading cause of early death in middle- and high-income countries and number two overall. Some have suggested that these younger generations may be the first in our history to have a shorter lifespan than that of their parents, because of what they're putting in their mouths. People in rapidly developing countries are at much greater risk of type 2 diabetes, obesity and heart disease, possibly because of their history of being undernourished. Their systems are wired to retain more energy from the diet as fat. This relates to what we discussed earlier – that children born to undernourished mothers are more prone to weight gain. The projections from official sources are that 70 per cent of the burden of type 2 diabetes will fall to those in these countries, particularly because of the rapid changes they have experienced in their diets.

India is an excellent example of this nutritional transition. Rates of overweight and obesity have tripled in India since 1990 when the government opened its trade borders to multinational corporations such as Coca-Cola and PepsiCo, which are investing billions of dollars in expanding into the Indian market. Since 2010, sales of packaged foods have increased nearly 140 per cent, and sales of junk food more than 80 per cent. As the impact of the changes in the food supply spread to even rural and remote areas in India, it's expected that more than 120 million people will have type 2 diabetes by 2040. While many policies have been proposed to address the growing predominance of processed foods and the associated rising tsunami of illness, such as limiting the sale of junk foods near schools, reducing marketing of such foods to children, and introducing nutrition labelling and junk food taxes, all have been vociferously opposed by the food industry, and such changes are mostly yet to take place.

The recommendations from the World Health Organization (WHO)

The WHO, in recognition of the scale and urgency of the threats to global health, called for large-scale and integrated policy action at regional, national and local levels at their emergency meeting in 2011. These include laws, regulations, taxes and subsidies affecting aspects of the food system, as well as population monitoring systems and nutrition promotion strategies. Interventions such as restricting the marketing of unhealthy foods and drinks, taxation and better nutrition labelling on food packages are considered essential elements in the attempt to turn the tide, yet the pushback from industry has been and continues to be extraordinary. The WHO also made heads of government responsible for the urgent and profound changes that needed to happen to address the food industry, yet very little has fundamentally changed since then. The vested interests are just too great.

As just one example, the food and beverage industry is believed to have spent an estimated €1 billion to win a lobbying battle against the introduction of traffic-light labelling (red, amber, green) on packaged foods in the European Union. Research also shows that Big Food spends approximately 30 times more on advertisements for junk food than governments spend on healthy food advertising. And they wouldn't do that if advertising wasn't very effective in getting people to eat their products. Following in the footsteps of the tobacco industry, they've also been remarkably effective in imparting a message that any legislative changes to the availability, marketing and cost of junk foods are evidence of a 'nanny state' that should be resisted. I don't think members of the general public who tout this line recognise that this idea comes directly from the industry that stands to benefit from it. Industry also funds research 'showing' that obesity comes from a lack of exercise rather than diet, or that sugar-sweetened beverages don't make a big contribution to the obesity epidemic. Non-industry-funded research tells us, however, that the real culprit is the changes to the food system, with increases in the quantity of available food, and especially of industrialised foods with added fats, sugars, salt and flavours – all designed to make us want more of them.

Campaigns in Australia

In Australia, the recent 'Tipping the Scales' campaign by the Obesity Policy Coalition requested urgent government action to address the serious obesity problem we're facing. It called for eight actions, including advertising restrictions, mandatory health ratings on packaging, a 20 per cent levy on sugary drinks, the setting of food reformulation targets, better monitoring of diet and physical activity guidelines, the funding of public health campaigns, and an active transport strategy. They also called for the establishment of a national obesity taskforce.

And yet both sides of politics have rejected the calls, particularly for a tax on sweet drinks, despite the incredible scale of our problem. Why? Because of the very large industry players that would be affected by a drop in sales of these drinks. The Australian Food and Grocery Council, Australian Beverages Council, Canegrowers, the Australian Sugar Milling Council, the Australian Sugar Industry Alliance, the Australian Association of National Advertisers, the Australian Industry Group, and the Australasian Association of Convenience Stores all formed a partnership to lobby to keep the policy off the table. The key tactics of these sorts of industry groups are to downplay the data concerning the health impacts of these food products, while also framing the debate around personal choices (the nanny state argument) and the impact of higher costs on poorer communities. Just as the tobacco industry has done for so long. They of course neglect the massive costs to individuals, communities and the wider public purse of the health impacts arising from these food products. They also ignore research, such as the findings of the WHO Collaborating Centre for Obesity Prevention, which estimated a saving to the Australian public purse of close to $2 billion over the lifespan of the current population with the introduction of a 20 per cent tax on sugar-sweetened drinks.

On the other hand, unlike tobacco, food is a highly complex 'product', and big-stick legislation can inadvertently get it wrong. An example of this is the saturated-fat tax that was introduced in Denmark in 2011 but repealed less than a year later because of the recognition that it wasn't working. Danes were going across their borders to purchase their unhealthy snacks, and the administrative burden on producers was considered untenable. The tax also affected unprocessed ingredients such as milk and cheese. These, particularly unprocessed cheeses including feta, goat's cheese, parmesan cheese, blue cheese and the like, are healthy products in moderation, and sources of nutrition as well as bacteria and their metabolites. This is a good example of where legislative approaches need to be nuanced or aimed at a single culprit.

An excellent model of 'single-culprit' approaches is the tax on sugar-sweetened beverages (such as fizzy drinks), either in place or proposed now in many countries around the world. The initial data from countries that have had such a tax in place for a while now suggest that these taxes do act to reduce consumption. For example, in Mexico where a soda tax was introduced in 2014, sales of sugary drinks have declined by at least 17 per cent. In another study of several low-income areas of San Francisco, where the United States' first soda tax was introduced in 2014, reported consumption of sugary drinks fell more than 20 per cent in the first four months of the tax, while it went up in neighbouring communities without the tax. People in the area with the tax also reported drinking more water, suggesting that they were replacing these sugary drinks with a healthier (and cheaper!) option.

In general, it's understood that a 10 per cent tax leads to 10 per cent reduction in purchase, but other research has suggested that taxes on unhealthy foods would need to increase prices by at least 20 per cent to have any impact on obesity rates. If we again look to the tobacco industry as a parallel, the reductions in smoking rates that we have now achieved in most Western countries took decades and required a large number of different approaches, including taxation, school interventions, clean indoor air regulations, agricultural initiatives, advertising campaigns, medical care initiatives, community mobilisation and political action. In the United States, tobacco prices have risen at least 50 per cent since the end of last century, and this has had a dramatic effect on smoking rates. In Australia, the tax on cigarettes is approximately 400 per cent, so a 20 per cent tax on junk food is well worth considering in my view. A comprehensive evaluation by colleagues of mine in 2010, the Assessing Cost-Effectiveness in Prevention (ACE-Prevention) report, concluded that a 10 per cent tax on 'junk' food would be a highly cost-effective strategy for improving physical health outcomes in Australia. Certainly, given that Australians get more of their added sugars from sweetened drinks each year than they get from all the cakes, chocolate, ice cream, biscuits, pastries, muffins, yoghurts, cereal, scones and sweets combined, targeting sugar-sweetened beverages with taxes makes very good sense!

However, to be truly effective, taxes need to be paired with subsidies for whole foods and a range of other initiatives, including legislative restrictions to industry marketing and to the foods that can be sold in schools, hospitals, leisure centres and other government-funded, community-based settings. If we consider the intergenerational transmission of disease, and the impact of the metabolic health of parents on neurodevelopmental outcomes in their children, it's clear that we need to put every strategy and effort in place to prevent young people becoming obese and unhealthy in the first place. For this reason, it's essential to ensure that children are being given the right nutrition messages everywhere they go.

The importance of education

One final important point: many health researchers believe that one of the most effective and cost-effective ways to prevent poor lifestyles choices and their health consequences is to support access to education. A very convincing body of evidence shows that the higher a person's educational attainment, the better their health over time. More-educated people smoke less, are less likely to drink excessively, weigh less and exercise more. They're more likely to listen to and act on the advice of medical and public-health professionals and die later than those with less education as a result. Even right back at the start of life, children who have access to quality preschools are less likely to end up as smokers, are less likely to drink excessively as they become adults and have better mental health and overall health as they age. So investing in quality child care and public education is another important strategy for policymakers to put a dent in the current health disaster. And of course, having access to kitchen gardens and cooking and nutrition programs in schools is essential. More of that below.

What can parents do?

Less than *half a per cent* of Australian children eat enough vegetables and legumes for health. Children and adolescents in Australia get roughly *40 per cent* of their average daily calories from extremely processed junk foods, such as fizzy drinks, chicken nuggets, packaged crisps, doughnuts, and instant noodles and soups. A single frozen slushy drink – so popular with young people – can contain an entire week's worth of sugar in *one hit*. Rates of obesity in children have *tripled* since the 1970s. The younger generation may have a *shorter lifespan* than their parents because of what they are putting in their mouths. Unhealthy diet is now the *leading cause of early death* across middle- and high-income countries, and number two overall. It's expected to cost the global community at least *US$30 trillion* over the next decade or so. The scale of this disaster is mind-boggling. And yet, to date, no country anywhere in the world has made even a dent in its obesity epidemic, which is the most visible indicator of the disastrous changes to our food systems.

If obesity were an acute illness, such as an influenza epidemic, government agencies all over the world would be ramping up every effort, making every resource available, and treating it as the disastrous and massive public health emergency that it is. But because it has crept up insidiously, over many decades and many, many political cycles, and (mainly) because of the many billions of dollars and vested interests involved, politicians and policymakers everywhere are largely refusing to act. We've discussed this. But there's another aspect to this that I believe is just as worrying: the fact that the general public and, in particular, parents are not 'seeing' the scale of the disaster either.

Parents need to act

We know, from many studies, that parents simply don't perceive their children to be overweight, even if they objectively are. Overweight and obesity are now so common as to be normalised. And parents don't like to believe that there's any problem with the status quo. They have – in very many cases – been successfully brainwashed by the Big Food industry to associate junk and processed foods with 'treats' and 'family time' and 'summertime'. These are examples of the industry's very clever tactics to encourage people to pair the idea of food treats, mentally and emotionally, with happy, wholesome events and images. Parents also see what other children eat at home or at school and start to consider it normal. They give in to the pressure from their children for packaged snacks in lunchboxes. This feels like nurturing. And they're time- and energy-poor, which compounds everything. This is why convenience foods were such a bit hit when they first went mainstream back in the middle of last century: to be able to open a packet rather than cook a meal from scratch – what a revolution! And parents seem reluctant to give this up.

I read, just this morning, the results of an online survey of Australian parents where they were offered a series of choices for the foods that could be made available at their children's school canteen – starting with healthy foods, but then adding fewer healthy and more unhealthy foods. So, for example, snack options started with only fruit, but then added in popcorn, pretzels, cakes, muffins, muesli bars and ice creams, then chips and bags of sweets. Amazingly (to me), the largest proportion of parents – nearly 45 per cent – were in favour of offering the full gamut of foods, including all the junk foods. Only 12 per cent of the parents chose the option where the school canteens would only have healthy food options (sandwiches, wraps, salads and fruit).

If we want to normalise whole, nutritious food, and we want our children to learn to make good food choices as a matter of course so that their bodies and brains can grow optimally – and do the same for their own children when they become parents – it's critical that we start to tackle our children's food environment, and the implicit messages it sends, right from the start. I believe that educational institutions could be leading the charge in setting the best examples and supporting healthy eating as the norm for children.

Schools need to act

Schools are in a unique position in that children spend a very large proportion of their most formative years there. Some schools have wonderful programs where children can grow and then prepare and eat their own vegetables, where they're taught to appreciate fresh, whole foods and to learn about the importance of these to their health. But such programs are ad hoc in most cases – it depends on the school and its parent population, whether or not they prioritise this, and want to or can raise the funds needed for such programs. Many of the schools in the most disadvantaged areas, where there is most need, don't have such resources, and these programs aren't funded by governments. Given the massive scale of the problems we face, I believe that they should be a priority. But there's no point teaching children to grow, cook and appreciate whole foods and then making ultra-processed, high-fat, high-sugar foods available in canteens and vending machines. Or allowing these sorts of foods to be sold close to schools, where children can access them before, after and even during the school day.

A wonderful piece appeared in the *New York Times* recently about Rahul Verma, who in 2010 filed a public interest lawsuit in the Delhi High Court seeking a ban on the sale of junk food and soft drinks in and around schools across India. Although his lawsuit has not (yet) been successful, it has prompted the courts to order the government of India to develop guidelines regarding junk food. Again, however, the pushback from industry has been vociferous, and most of the suggested changes are yet to take place. In Australia, even prolonged and energetic campaigns by communities to restrict fast-food outlets from setting up in particular towns or near schools have repeatedly failed, largely because they require bureaucratically challenging changes to planning laws that are vigorously fought by big business. That doesn't mean we shouldn't keep trying. We need to be energetic and effective advocates for the health of our children. And of course, we need to set the very best examples in our homes, right from the start of life.

We need to start early

Children are primed to like sweet tastes more than bitter, sour or more complex tastes. So they need to be 'trained' from the beginning to make good choices, and the eating of healthy, whole foods must be normalised. Children need at least six exposures to a new taste to accept it and develop a liking for it. Give babies a wide range of vegetables, fruits and other (age-appropriate) whole foods from the start, and don't give up if they reject them at first. And definitely don't give in to the idea that it's better for children to have 'something' rather than not eating at all. Children won't starve themselves, and if you have a pantry and fridge full of healthy foods, where packaged and unhealthy foods are absent, it's much more likely that they'll grow up making good choices.

You can use fun approaches like making fruits and vegetables different shapes or having competitions to see who can eat the rainbow. Get children used to water as their standard drink; you can add lemon or mint to enhance the flavour or use ice cubes with fruit pieces. Make bottles of frozen water with these sorts of additions for kids to take to school – they'll be thawed by lunchtime. It's about setting an example and making these sorts of choices the default. And don't forget to turn off the television at mealtimes and discourage snacking while watching TV. Couch snacking is a major contributor to overeating. I also think it's really helpful and important to get children involved in the planning and preparation of meals. They'll be far more likely to eat a meal that they've chosen or contributed to.

One very important thing I should point out is that many people regard junk food and unhealthy diets for children as solely an issue in economically disadvantaged families. While those with less money and education are particularly affected by the obesogenic environment, the fact is that people right across the socioeconomic spectrum are eating very badly. Indeed, I have many highly educated and well-off friends and colleagues whose cupboards are full of packaged foods, and whose children eat processed cereals, white bread and rice, pastries, biscuits, ice creams, chips and the like every day. As I said, this way of eating has become normalised, and it has many drivers, including the particularly effective way these foods interact with the reward systems in the brain. This is why it's a long, slow process to change things around. But they can be changed.

Getting it right at home

One of the great pleasures of my job is the opportunity to meet fascinating people from many fields. One particularly interesting person I had met and got to know is Carolyn Creswell, the founder and owner of Carman's Muesli. She built this company from scratch and it's now highly successful, selling muesli products in many countries. I had lunch with Carolyn one day and she told me about how she and her family had gradually made the transition to a healthy diet.

She told me that when she was growing up, the diet in her family home was typically Anglo-Australian: white-bread sandwiches with margarine, meat with some tired peas and potatoes for dinner, and soft drinks, doughnuts, chips and biscuits in the cupboard. She didn't know how to cook and wasn't interested in learning. At 18, however, she became involved with Carman's and started to realise that so many processed foods had additives, such as emulsifiers and flavourings. Around the same time, she started shopping for her grandmother and noted that *her* shopping list consisted of mainly whole and fresh foods rather than packaged foods. Her grandma would say, 'Food should come from the kitchen and not from the chemist.' Carolyn started to become more focused on nutrition and, in particular, what made her feel good (and bad). She went through a period of low mood and started to make the connection between her diet and her mood and sense of wellbeing. This led her to learn more about nutrition and to take more care when choosing her foods, particularly once she had her own family.

She now believes she has the balance right in her home and follows the 80/20 rule – 80 per cent healthy whole foods and 20 per cent 'treats'. But these treats are generally homemade and not overly processed. She doesn't have processed meats in the house, nor is her cupboard stocked with chips or biscuits and the like. Importantly, she has worked with her children to help them to discover their food preferences and to teach them to cook, so that they can have some agency over their diets. They do a big cook-up together on Sundays, choosing from different healthy recipes, so that they have food prepared for the week. Carolyn's is a story that highlights how positive dietary changes can be made, even if the diet you grew up with left you with little knowledge of how to eat well.

Similarly, my kids learnt to eat a full range of whole vegetables and fruit right from the beginning. I remember Ivy sitting up in her highchair scoffing down lentil dhal with her hands when she was less than a year old. It made a big mess, which I'm sure increased the appeal. She and her sister used to fight over the broccoli (trees)! We didn't have much money when they were young as I was studying, but I would still try to make sure that they had a big plate of cut fruit and some nuts after school, and would always make them something we called 'magic purple potion'. I had an old juicer that I'd got from the op shop; I would cut up fresh beetroot, carrot, pineapple and apple, and juice them with some lemon juice. The kids loved it. Nowadays there are wonderful contraptions that do this far more easily, and without losing the valuable pulp (fibre).

My kids always ate healthy meals at home because that's what they were given. Not to say that I didn't make it easy for myself; one of my go-to meals in the evening was a big pile of mashed sweet potato (skins left on of course) covered in steamed spinach and topped with tinned sardines and a bit of soy sauce. That might sound gross, but it was really tasty as well as quick and easy. My husband Rob made a great vegie and tuna pasta with tinned tuna and beans. He also made a legendary spaghetti bolognese with lentils or beans and loads of vegies. We both made a lot of soups – it was quick and easy to add lots of vegies (sometimes frozen, sometimes fresh) to tinned tomatoes or vegetable stock, add some lentils or beans and a stock cube, and have it with a lovely slice of wholegrain toast with olive oil. Fish soup was also an easy one – adding some blue grenadier (which is cheap) to tinned tomato, onion and garlic, rice, then adding lemon juice and spinach at the end. Yum.

Both my girls are passionate about good food and love to cook. They now share a flat and take turns making lovely meals for each other and their friends. They're great examples of what happens when whole foods are made the default from the start. It goes without saying that we didn't have chips, chocolate, ice creams, sweetened drinks and other such snack foods in the house. I have *zero* willpower, so why try to resist temptation when it's so much easier just to avoid it?

Is there any good news?

I'm happy to say that there are hints that things are starting to improve at the population level. Sales of sugar-sweetened fizzy drinks and the big fast-food chains are gradually declining, and industry is starting to respond to consumer preferences for healthier food options. A recently released survey of food manufacturers worldwide reported that they reformulated more than 180,000 products in 2016, primarily focusing on reducing sugar and salt contents, but also adding more whole grains and vitamins to products. At the same time, healthier versions of fast-food chains have increased in number and popularity in many Western countries, such as chains focused on Mexican foods, which are full of beans, salads and whole grains. Of course, it's still possible to overeat these – or eat the less healthy version where you smother your meal with cheese and sour cream and wash it down with a fizzy drink – but choosing wisely allows for the occasional convenience of prepared foods without the health impact. In our house, we love prepared sushi rolls with fish and avocado or Indian curries with lentils and vegetables for our takeaway treats.

Other positive changes in the marketplace that I'm starting to see are based on 'nudge' theory, which was developed by Richard Thaler and recently won him the Nobel Prize in Economics. The basis of this idea is to make subtle changes to the environment that don't penalise people for bad choices, but rather make it easier for them to make good choices without them even being aware of it. A key example of this theory in action is in major supermarkets, where nudge theory has been previously used to encourage people to make unhealthy purchasing decisions, for example by putting confectionery at the checkout, within easy reach of children. But it's increasingly being used to drive healthier choices.

In Australia, a large supermarket chain, recognising the increased concern in the community regarding obesity and diabetes, has begun to change its checkouts so they have healthier snacks on offer. It also offers fresh fruit, free, to children to snack on while their parents are shopping. Happily, people's shopping baskets are changing for the better; fruit has jumped from tenth to second on the list of bestselling grocery items in Australia in the past decade, while the purchase of sweets, fizzy drinks and chocolates has declined. This is great news.

All these sorts of positive changes are driven not by politicians or government legislators, but rather by changing consumer preferences. Politicians and business don't take action unless it's clear that the majority (or at least a powerful minority) of the community want them to. For this reason, it's essential that we, as citizens, provide pressure with our voices, our votes and our wallets.

Key facts

- There's increasing interest in integrating diet, exercise and other behavioural changes into the treatment of mental health conditions, but there's a lack of training in diet and exercise for medical students.
- People with serious mental illnesses (SMIs) die up to 20 years earlier than people without such illnesses.
- Interventions to help people with their diet, exercise habits, smoking and body weight can have a big benefit for health outcomes in people with SMIs.
- Clinical dietitians or nutritionists are best placed to conduct dietary interventions, as they're trained in helping people to make healthy changes to their diet.
- Support for access to clinical dietitians for everyone with mental health issues is likely to be a highly cost-effective way to improve outcomes for individuals and the population.
- Getting children used to a wide variety of whole foods from an early age and making sure your house is 'health-friendly' is essential in setting up good eating habits from the start of life.

- Big Food has a strong vested interest in maintaining the unhealthy status quo, and is very effective at pushing back against taxes and other legislative changes that might affect its profits. Nonetheless, there are positive signs that things are changing for the better.
- We, as citizens, need to apply pressure in any way we can to ensure that the next generation has a much healthier food environment – and thus better health outcomes – than what we have now.

11

Myths and hits

I suspect that no other topic has given rise to as many myths, contradictory messages and as much misinformation as nutrition. A lot of the reasons for this relate to what we discussed earlier: the methodological issues that make nutrition research so challenging. But the other thing about diet and nutrition is that everyone eats, and most people hold strong opinions about what is healthy or not healthy based on their own experiences, that of their friends and family, and – of course – their cultural traditions.

But people also get information from 'experts' who can present information in a way that can be heavily biased or misleading, based on their own personal beliefs. Even medical practitioners can get it wrong, particularly if they're not trained in research and don't have a clear understanding of how to interpret research evidence correctly. In fact, medical practitioners are often the worst offenders, as they rely on their clinical experiences to form opinions and make recommendations, which we know is a very flawed approach (remember Chapter 5?).

Many people also have a financial interest in promoting a particular diet, food, or nutrition product. Certainly, Big Food has a very strong vested interest in confusing people about what is healthy or isn't healthy. For all these reasons, it may be useful for me to set out here what we do (and don't) know about popular topics, ideas and sources of debate in nutrition and Nutritional Psychiatry.

Is red meat good or bad for us?

You might remember, when I was talking about my PhD, that I had, unexpectedly, identified a third dietary pattern that was high in fruits and salads plus fish, tofu, beans, nuts, yoghurt, and red wine, and that this pattern showed a slight tendency to be associated with more, rather than less, depression in women. I was quite surprised and very interested to see this because it clearly looks like a pretty healthy dietary pattern, and I would have guessed that it would be protective against depression. At first I thought that it might be explained by the tendency for some people with anxiety (which very often co-occurs with depression) to be obsessed with eating a healthy diet (reverse causality). But when you're a scientist, getting a result that's the opposite of your hypothesis can be just as interesting or exciting as having your hypotheses confirmed. So I went on to dig a bit deeper.

As part of my PhD, as well as investigating overall diet, I also looked at the dietary intake (not supplements) of individual nutrients and food groups and their relationship to mental health. I know I said at the start that this approach was problematic because it didn't consider overall diet, but I was doing a PhD and it needed to be thorough! I also had a few pet hypotheses of my own that I wanted to test, particularly in relation to animal foods. This is because I'd been brought up as a vegetarian by my strictly vegetarian father and had been somewhat indoctrinated into the idea that foods coming from animals were not good for health. Personally speaking, I'd always felt very ambivalent about animal foods – particularly the way animals are treated as part of industrialised agriculture, as well as the environmental impacts of meat production. For this reason, although I wasn't still a strict vegetarian, I'd been mainly vegetarian for most of my life and very rarely ate red meat or poultry (although I did eat some fish).

Because of these personal beliefs and lifelong practices, I was very interested to test the hypothesis that women with a higher intake of animal foods (meat, poultry, dairy, eggs) would have worse mental health. When I investigated this, however, I did see a very clear relationship between animal food consumption and mental health, but not in the direction I expected.

Women who scored higher on animal food intakes were, in fact, 20–30 per cent *less* likely to have a history of depressive or anxiety disorder. What could this mean? I wanted to delve deeper, so I started to look at the data in even more detail. What I noticed was that the particularly healthy ('modern') food pattern that had shown a hint of being associated with more rather than less depression in my PhD study was low in red meat. I also noted that there were quite a few studies showing that vegetarians are more likely to have mental health problems such as depression or anxiety. But it had always been assumed that the vegetarianism arose as a *result* of the person's mental health. When I looked at our animal food group in detail, it was the red meat component of the animal group that was strongly associated with less depression and anxiety in the women – eggs, dairy and poultry didn't show much of a relationship with any mental health outcome, although there was a hint that processed meat was associated with worse mental health.

Wanting to understand further, I divided the women up into three groups according to the Australian dietary guidelines for red meat intake. The recommendations are for three to four small (65–100 gram – palm-sized, in other words) servings of unprocessed red meat (beef and lamb) per week, so I grouped women according to whether they consumed roughly that amount or less or more than that amount. And then, because of the link between vegetarianism and mental health, I actually excluded the 20 or so women who consumed no meat or poultry at all, and restricted the investigation to low, moderate, or high red meat intake.

Finally, because people who eat a lot of meat may also eat lots of healthy foods, such as vegetables, or they might eat lots of unhealthy foods alongside their red meat, I also took into account the women's overall diet quality. And what we found was intriguing.

Compared to women consuming the recommended amount of red meat, those women who were eating either less *or* more than the recommended amount per week were roughly twice as likely to have a clinical depressive or anxiety disorder. This meant that the relationship was what we call U-shaped. And it was very consistent; we even saw this pattern of association when we looked at the women's psychological symptoms (in other words, not just clinical mental disorders).

We published these findings in 2012 and, needless to say, they created a lot of interest in the media. Our study had come hot on the heels of another very large study of more than 20,000 people from the United States suggesting that red meat consumption increases the risk of early death, which had also been extensively covered in the news. So why did we find something so different?

There could be quite a few reasons, but one possibility I think is that meat in Australia is very different from US meat. In the

United States, 99 per cent of all beef comes from feedlots, where cattle are raised in captivity and fed a diet high in grains. This means that they have a very different fatty acid profile from cattle that are raised eating grass in pastures – the way most meat in Australia is raised. Grain-fed beef has more omega-6 fatty acids, which are linked to inflammation, whereas grass-fed beef is higher in long-chain omega-3 fatty acids – the ones that have been linked to improved mental health. Studies in healthy Australian men comparing vegetarians to meat-eaters showed lower omega-3 fatty acid concentrations in vegetarians and vegans. Of course, there are other possible explanations for our findings, such as not being able to measure fully how people who eat a lot of, or not very much, red meat differ from others in terms of the rest of their diet or other health behaviours. There is also the established link between higher anxiety and restrictive dietary behaviours, and it's possible that certain personality factors may predispose to both vegetarianism and veganism and mental health problems. But certainly, our findings did add to the increasing numbers of studies linking vegetarianism or low meat intake to poorer mental health, as well as too much meat being noxious to health.

It's probably worth pointing out that, while I'm largely vegetarian for ethical reasons, I do encourage my daughters to eat small amounts of red meat at least a couple of times a week. Given my family history (and, thus, theirs) and the many anecdotal reports I've heard from doctors and other health professionals about the number of young female vegetarians they see in their clinics with severe depression, I'm not going to take any chances, particularly while my daughters are menstruating and coming into their childbearing years. However, I do support them to source meat from farms with ethical animal husbandry practices. The extra cost is offset by them eating smaller portions. And they always pair their meat with plenty of vegetables and high fibre legumes, which is important to reduce the risk of cancer associated with red meat intake (the fibre pushes the meat through the bowel more quickly and the antioxidants in the vegetables also counteract the small amount of DNA damage that red meat inflicts).

Is dairy good for us?

Dairy foods, including milk, yoghurt and cheese, are considered an essential part of a healthy, balanced diet, as they contain many vitamins and minerals, as well as protein. Several serves a day are generally recommended for a range of health benefits, including improved bone mineral density, cardiovascular health, prevention of some forms of cancer and even weight maintenance (we're talking sensible portions without added sugars here – not ice cream, processed cheeses, flavoured milks, sweetened yoghurts and all the other junk you'll find on the supermarket shelves).

These recommendations are based on research evidence, but it's important to note that some of that evidence is quite contradictory. For example, although dairy foods are recommended, on the basis of their calcium content, to prevent osteoporosis, some studies link increased milk consumption with a *higher* risk of fractures. This is not the only health endpoint that has contradictory findings with regard to dairy foods: we found in our large GOS cohort that women who drank the equivalent of a glass of milk or more a day were at increased risk of clinical depression, but we only saw this in women who were past menopause. In younger women, there was no relationship between dairy intake and mental health. In contrast, another study of older Japanese people found that low-fat (but not full-fat) dairy consumption was associated with lower levels of depressive symptoms. In the main, however, studies have either found no link between dairy foods and depression or inconsistent and conflicting relationships.

A number of aspects of dairy foods might explain these inconsistent findings, particularly with regard to mental health. First, full (saturated) fat dairy foods have been linked in some studies with poorer cognition and cognitive decline and, as we've already discussed, high-saturated-fat intake is associated with a range of negative effects on the brain and gut. On the other hand, a recent systematic review concluded that dairy may *reduce* the risk of cognitive decline by helping with weight loss, improving glucose regulation, and reducing inflammation and blood pressure. Dairy increases something called insulin-like growth factor-1, which has also been linked to depression, and dairy is also a primary dietary source of something called D-galactose, which generates oxidative stress in the body. As we've discussed, oxidative stress appears to be both a cause and consequence of mental health problems. The whey in dairy, however, provides cysteine, which is essential in the production of glutathione, the brain's main natural antioxidant. Dairy foods also supply tryptophan, which is a precursor to serotonin production. Thus there are both potential health risks and benefits to aspects of dairy that might explain conflicting research findings.

A1 versus A2 milk

We at the Food & Mood Centre are currently exploring another intriguing aspect of milk in a randomised, controlled trial in women. This relates to the major protein found in milk called casein, and in particular beta-casein.

The original form of beta-casein is considered to be the A2 beta-casein. A natural mutation occurred in genes coding for beta-casein in European dairy herds thousands of years ago, which resulted the A1 beta-casein variant; this is structurally different from the original A2 beta-casein. Subsequently, this mutation was passed on to other breeds, gradually making A1 beta-casein more common in milk around the world. Most of the European herds (Holstein Friesian cattle) produce milk containing A1 beta-casein as well as A2, while purebred Asian and African herds produce milk containing only A2 beta-casein (Guernsey, Jersey cattle). In the United States, the Holstein breed makes up 92 per cent of the dairy cows, whereas the Guernsey breed makes up only about 1 per cent. In Australia, the Holstein breed makes up to 78 per cent of the dairy cows. In fact, the large majority of dairy in Western countries contains the A1 protein as well as the A2 protein, in a roughly 1:1 ratio. Goats, sheep and other milk-producing animals (including humans!), however, still produce milk containing only A2 beta-casein.

When digested, the A1 type of beta-casein, but not A2 beta-casein, produces a bioactive peptide (short protein) called beta-casomorphin 7 (BCM-7). BCM-7 is a peptide with opioid properties and can act in a similar way to morphine. The A1 beta-casein protein variant has been shown in animal research to promote gastrointestinal inflammation and increased levels of pro-inflammatory cytokines, and to reduce glutathione levels, all of which are implicated in depression. Even just one cup of milk containing A1 beta-casein may produce enough BCM-7 to have pharmacological effects.

Interestingly, countries differ in the proportion of their cow herds with the A1 variation or the original A2 gene, and this appears to be linked to the prevalence of some diseases. For example, most Scandinavian countries (Norway, Sweden, Denmark and Finland) have high proportions of cattle with the A1 genetic profile, whereas – because of its geographical isolation from the mainland – Iceland has lower A1 proportions. There are lower rates of type 1 diabetes in Iceland compared to the Scandinavian countries, and the recent increase in the incidence of type 1 diabetes in the Scandinavian countries is not apparent in Iceland, despite the genetic and cultural similarities between these populations. Type 1 diabetes is an autoimmune disease, and elevated levels of antibodies to A1 beta-casein have been found in people newly diagnosed with type 1 diabetes. Another study examining the per capita consumption of A1 beta-casein across 20 different countries also showed a strong correlation with type 1 diabetes as well as with ischemic heart disease. There's also evidence linking dairy proteins to mental disorders. More than 90 per cent of people with schizophrenia and 86 per cent of those with autism were found to have antibodies to BCM-7, while new data suggests a suppression of immune responses to dairy proteins in depressed people.

For all of these reasons, we're currently running a trial that compares the consumption of conventional dairy, which contains the A1 and A2 beta-casein protein variants, with dairy containing only A2. We'll examine a number of health endpoints, including psychological distress, depression, anxiety, stress and cognition in women who will be randomly assigned to either type of dairy products for four months. We'll also examine a number of biological markers in blood, as well as measures of gut health (microbiota, symptoms, leaky gut). This study is easier than some to perform because the two variants of dairy products are identical in taste and appearance, so the study will be truly blinded. It will be very interesting to see whether there are differences between the two groups of women on any of these endpoints at the end of the study.

Fermented dairy foods

It's important to note that, as with many foods, the fermentation process can change the health properties and composition of dairy foods. When dairy foods are fermented to yield products such as yoghurt, kefir and cheese (not the processed rubbery stuff, but 'real' cheese), this process – driven by lactic acid bacteria – produces a myriad of components with many important health properties. In addition to these functions, these bacteria may also impart beneficial health functions such as reducing inflammation and strengthening the immune system and vitamin production. Personally, I would crawl through the Kalahari Desert for blue cheese and I'm quite addicted to yoghurt and kefir. I make my own kefir at home – it's very easy and inexpensive.

Are 'paleo' diets the answer?

The 'Paleolithic diet' has become very popular with many in the community in recent years. The fundamental premise of the Paleolithic diet is that, because the human genome takes thousands of years to evolve and adapt to a changing environment, we're still genetically Stone Agers and thus optimised to eat a Stone Age diet. Proponents suggest that it's essential to cut grains, legumes and dairy foods from the diet, as we are not equipped (genetically) to digest them properly.

This idea was very influential when it was first proposed, and it makes intuitive sense; indeed, when I was starting out in research, this idea strongly influenced my dietary choices for a while. The theory is, however, fundamentally flawed, although we only understood this recently. This is because, while our genomes take aeons to evolve, our gut microbiota – which are our primary adaptive 'organ' – change rapidly in response to changing environmental conditions and exposures. As just one example, the gut microbiota of Japanese people has particular bugs that are good at digesting seaweed. Our microbiota can start to adapt to new foods within hours, and this means that humans have been successfully able to thrive in many highly diverse parts of the planet with very different available food sources.

Having said that, studies examining Palaeolithic nutrition and existing hunter-gatherer populations tell us that dietary intakes of micronutrients and fibre for early humans may have been up to ten times those of modern humans, due to the amount, diversity and composition of wild plant foods known to be eaten by hunter-gatherers. Of course, carbohydrates in the diet came almost exclusively from fruits and vegetables, and there were no easy sources of simple sugars (apart from the occasional honey treat, if you managed to survive the bees). So they avoided the refined carbohydrates and sugary drinks (as well as alcohol and tobacco) that are making us so sick. Foods were also low in sodium and very high in potassium, which offers a far better balance for health. The meat people ate would have been a very different (and healthier) 'beast' compared to the meats we now have access to from intensive farming methods. Finally, estimates suggest that humans evolved to consume a diet consisting of equal parts omega-6 and omega-3 fatty acids. In stark contrast, the current ratio in Western diets is 10–20:1. Given what we know about the importance of omega-3 fatty acids to our health, the fact that this balance is so out of whack now may be a driver of disease, particularly inflammation.

So should you drop the grains, dairy and legumes from your diet just because cave people didn't apparently eat these? No, not at all.

Are grains and gluten really so bad?

Several high-profile books of late have pointed the finger at grains, and wheat in particular, as the culprit for virtually every health problem under the sun – obesity, type 2 diabetes, other metabolic disorders, heart disease, asthma, autism, irritable bowel syndrome, other serious bowel disorders, right through to serious mental and brain disorders such as dementia. But the evidence for these contentions doesn't hold up well to scientific scrutiny so far. The main issue that really muddies the waters is the quality of carbohydrates that people consume in Western countries, particularly the United States. Many people report a benefit from reducing their intake of carbohydrates (particularly grains), but this likely relates to the poor quality of carbohydrates in the modern food system, where cereals and breads are highly refined and processed, often with added sugars, and don't fit into the category of 'whole grains' in any shape or form (even those 'wholemeal' breads are often highly processed). Removing these from the diet will likely result in health benefits, but that doesn't mean that all wholegrains should be removed.

True wholegrains, including unprocessed and steel-cut oats (in other words, not the quick-cook types), barley, millet, buckwheat, rye, freekeh, quinoa, brown rice and the like, are important sources of phytochemicals, and many are also sources of beta-glucans, which help reduce inflammation. They are also very important sources of fermentable and non-fermentable fibre for our gut microbiota; many different types of fibre are important to the health of our gut and we need complex carbohydrates (fibre) from a diverse range of sources – including wholegrains, legumes, fruits and vegetables – to meet these needs (for some detail on dietary fibres and the gut, refer to the World Gastroenterology Organisation in the Sources). Research evidence tells us that a reduction in dietary carbohydrates for weight loss is associated with decreases in protective bacterial species in the bowel, as well as a decrease in antioxidant phenolic acids and other protective molecules.

Let's address some of the ideas that are put forward by some of the proponents in this field and see what stands up to scrutiny and what doesn't.

What role does non-coeliac gluten sensitivity play?

Gluten is a glycoprotein composed of two components: gliadin and glutenin. It's found mainly in wheat, rye and barley, and in a lower proportion in oats. Gluten is also commonly added to processed foods such as processed meats, cakes, biscuits, breads and sauces, and is even used as a drug-filler. People with coeliac disease, which is a severe autoimmune disorder, should avoid gluten completely, as even a tiny exposure damages the small intestine. But coeliac disease is quite rare, affecting only half to one per cent of the population. What is true is that the incidence of coeliac disease has risen dramatically in recent decades. This is likely due to a combination of factors, including increased awareness and diagnosis, but also – very possibly – the problems with the food system that impact on our gut health and thus our immune health.

On the other hand, people without coeliac disease very commonly now self-diagnose what is called non-coeliac gluten sensitivity (NCGS). These people find that the consumption of gluten-containing grains seems to cause gastrointestinal symptoms and IBS, and they get relief from these symptoms after removing gluten from their diets. These people are driving a very big increase in gluten-free diets throughout the Western world. But what is the evidence to date for this condition?

One study was carried out by my colleagues here in Australia specifically to examine whether the consumption of gluten could induce IBS symptoms. In this small double-blind, randomised, placebo-controlled trial of 34 people with self-reported NCGS, who were already on a gluten-free diet, participants were given foods (muffins and bread) that either contained gluten or were gluten-free for a period of six weeks. None of the participants or study assessors knew who was getting what. At the end of the study they found that nearly 70 per cent of the participants in the gluten group did report increased gut symptoms, compared to only 40 per cent of those getting the placebo products. This suggested that there were some people vulnerable to gluten itself, but it also showed evidence of the 'nocebo' response in those getting the gluten-free muffins.

It appears, however, that gluten itself may not necessarily be to blame. Gluten-containing grain products are commonly high in fermentable oligosaccharides, disaccharides and monosaccharides and polyols (FODMAPs), and for people with gut dysbiosis (very common) and symptoms of IBS, consumption of gluten-containing grains may cause gastrointestinal symptoms. When these colleagues again examined the effects of gluten and fructans (one type of FODMAP) separately in individuals with self-reported NCGS using a stricter trial methodology (they gave the participants all their food for the period of the study), they showed that it was actually the fructans that appeared to be responsible for people's gut symptoms, not gluten. In fact, they could not find evidence of NCGS in any of the people who had self-reported having it. That doesn't mean, however, that NCGS isn't 'real', but more that it's not nearly as common as believed. A more recent trial has just confirmed this finding. (Refer to J.R. Biesiekierski et al. in the Sources.)

More pertinent to our topic, these same researchers (who are considered leaders in this field) conducted another small study on 22 people with IBS who were on gluten-free diets, specifically to assess whether gluten would have an impact on symptoms of depression. And indeed, they found evidence that it did – those receiving the gluten-containing foods reported slightly worse symptoms of depression on average than those receiving placebo foods. So there is some evidence to suggest that gluten is a problem for a small subset of people. Given its limited size, however, this study needs to be replicated to be sure of the findings.

Similarly, there's some evidence that people with schizophrenia have higher levels of antibodies to gluten-containing foods. A meta-analysis reported that individuals with schizophrenia spectrum disorders had significantly elevated levels of five biomarkers of gluten sensitivity compared to healthy controls. The largest study so far, with 1401 schizophrenia patients and 900 healthy controls, found that the majority of patients had extremely high levels of antibodies to gluten and, in particular, higher levels of antibodies to anti-transglutaminase 6, which is a marker of coeliac disease. This is something found mainly in the brain and is related to neurological conditions, not intestinal diseases, which suggests the possibility that increased permeability of the blood–brain barrier in schizophrenia leads to an activation of immune cells.

Only a few intervention studies have been conducted in schizophrenia, however, and these have not been particularly rigorous from a scientific perspective; all of them had small sample sizes, almost all were open-label or single-blinded, and in half the studies, the intervention was not gluten-free only, but cereal-free and milk/casein-free as well. Two case studies have suggested that symptoms improved during a gluten-free phase and relapsed when gluten was reintroduced, but other studies showed no effect from removing gluten. As we discussed earlier, there's a high placebo/nocebo effect that needs to be accounted for with dietetic manipulations of this nature, such as gluten-free diets.

A recent comprehensive review on the topic concluded that there's insufficient evidence to recommend that people with severe mental disorders, such as mood disorders or schizophrenia, would benefit from avoiding gluten. We do think, however, that a small proportion of people with serious mental illnesses may have a food sensitivity that exacerbates their symptoms. Certainly, there's evidence that people with coeliac disease have an elevated risk of mental disorders, and that people with severe mental disorders, especially schizophrenia, might have an elevated risk of an abnormal immune response to gluten compared to the general population. However, they also have an increased risk of other immune-related bowel diseases, such as ulcerative colitis and Crohn's disease, as well as auto-immune diseases in general; thus, it remains unclear whether the immune response to gluten is more a result of the mental disorder than a cause, or due to a third factor (such as an impaired gut and immune system) that predisposes these people to both.

As we noted in Chapter 6, we're intending to run a pilot study of the ketogenic (very low-carbohydrate, high fat) diet in patients who are in hospital with psychotic illnesses, to see whether it might result in improvements in symptoms of psychosis. But in this study, it won't be possible for us to determine whether any effect on outcomes is a result of the ketogenic diet itself or the removal of potential allergens (such as grains) from the diet. This remains to be assessed in larger, more rigorous studies. We hope that our pilot study will provide initial data supporting grant applications to conduct these. In the meantime, scientific evidence on the potential role of gluten and other potential allergens in severe mental disorders remains scarce, and it's a topic that we believe needs further investigation.

Does avoiding grains lead to weight loss?

Previous research has suggested that diets that omit grains, which is one of the primary strategies of low-carb diets, lead to greater weight loss in the short term. The evidence also tells us, however, that over the longer term (say, a year) it doesn't offer any more weight loss benefit than other strategies but *is* harder to sustain. In nice bit of serendipity, in the week I'm writing this, a key intervention study has been published that really puts this question to bed. In this study – one of the best of its kind – the impact of low-fat versus low-carb diets was put to the test. This study was unusual in that it addressed many of the weaknesses of previous research in this area: it had a large sample size of more than 600 participants, whom it retained and tracked over a long period of time, and it very carefully assessed dietary compliance. What this study found was that both diets resulted in the same amount of weight loss over time.

Some people have suggested that wheat in particular leads to weight gain, but there's no good research evidence for this at this stage; weight gain comes from too much food, particularly of the wrong types. Processed foods, in particular, seem to be particularly successful in increasing body weight – possibly via their impact on the gut, as we discussed previously.

Do low-carbohydrate diets work for or against health?

In low-carbohydrate (LC) diets, the consumption of carbohydrates (coming from grains, rice, sweetened foods, starchy vegetables and sometimes even fruit) is restricted to less than 40–45 per cent of total energy intake, with some regimes (such as the ketogenic diet) restricting carbohydrates to as low as 5–10 per cent of the total energy per day. A large reduction in dietary carbohydrates, such as in the ketogenic diet, leads to depletion of glucose as the main source of energy in the body, resulting in the production of ketones that the body uses as an alternative energy source. This state of 'ketosis' means that fatty acids (including fats stored in the body) are used for energy, rather than carbohydrates. This sort of diet has become increasingly popular, as it can result in rapid weight loss and a reduction in appetite – and in a world of rampant obesity, this has obvious appeal.

There's very mixed evidence, however, regarding the long-term outcomes of LC diets. As noted above, the long-term benefits for weight loss are similar to other sorts of calorie-restricted diets, and there are very mixed findings regarding the long-term risks or benefits to health. In fact, there's quite extensive evidence from animal and human studies to show that over the long term, diets low in carbohydrates and high in animal proteins and/or fats result in early death and an increased risk of cardiovascular disease, cancer and other poor health outcomes.

Some evidence suggests that LC diets can result in health benefits in the short term, but in these studies where benefits to metabolic outcomes (improvements in cholesterol, triglycerides, blood pressure and so on) are shown, it's not clear whether they're simply a result of weight loss or of the diet itself. Similarly, in studies suggesting that reducing carbohydrates improves cardiometabolic health, it's believed that the benefit comes from removing refined carbohydrates from the diet, rather than the problem being carbohydrates themselves. If people get their carbohydrates from vegetables, fruits, legumes and real wholegrains, and *not* from refined and processed foods with added sweeteners, then the research evidence is overwhelming for the benefits of (complex) carbohydrates to health.

What I do see a lot of is people with an almost religious belief in the powers of LC or ketogenic-style diets to fix all cardiometabolic health problems. They feel that, because they've lost weight on these diets, this approach to eating is the best for health. While their belief is not backed by extensive scientific evidence at this stage, the research into the possible health benefits of different dietary approaches continues and is warranted. Not everyone will respond to the same diet in the same way – we know that people's microbiota differ enormously, and this has an impact on how they respond to different foods. Because of this, rigorous intervention studies will and should be conducted, and these may allow more personalised dietary recommendations in the future. I also suspect that adopting a LC diet in the short term is helpful for some people to kickstart their weight loss, reduce their blood glucose and retrain their palate, although, based on the research evidence, I personally wouldn't keep it up for more than a few weeks.

With regard to mental health, a handful of studies in over-weight or obese people have compared LC diets to low-fat or other types of diets; none of these have shown any differences to psychological health (depression, anxiety, mood or self-esteem). One very small study of 28 participants showed improvements in depression and self-esteem among people following a high-protein, LC diet compared to others following a low-protein, high-carbohydrate diet. However, a larger study of nearly 120 people showed *improvements* in psychological symptoms in those following a low-fat compared to a LC diet. As noted previously, a handful of case reports have found improvements in patients with schizophrenia following a ketogenic diet, and we urgently need properly conducted clinical trials to ascertain the benefits of this diet to mental health.

There is one new study that I think it important to mention. In this study, researchers from the University of North Carolina in the United States examined more than 11,000 women and their babies to see if there was a link between LC diets and birth defects. The reason they did this is because of the nutrient folate, which is very important in reducing the risk of spina bifida and other neural tube defects. Because women often don't eat enough green leafy vegetables, nuts, legumes and whole grains for sufficient folate in their diet, commercial cereals, breads and pasta are fortified with added folate. When women adopt LC diets, they then lose this important source of folate. What the researchers found was that women on LC diets were getting less than half the amount of folate in their diets as other women, and the risk of spina bifida and malformations of the brain and skull in their babies was increased by 30 per cent.

If we consider the importance of fibre to the gut and health, removing important sources of fibre (whole grains, legumes and starchy vegetables) from the diet is likely to be very problematic. As an example, a study in obese people showed that LC diets resulted in reductions in butyrate and butyrate-producing bacterial species. Butyrate is an important short chain fatty acid that is produced when bacteria ferment complex carbohydrates (fibre). LC diets tend to result in reduced intake of fibre and important dietary bioactive components (such as phytochemicals), and increased intake of saturated fat and protein from animal sources, all of which are linked to an increased risk of heart disease and mortality. In a review of four cohort studies involving more than 270,000 participants from multiple countries, long-term LC diets (5–26 years) were associated with an increased risk of early death. Similarly, in animal studies, we see that animals fed a LC diet lose weight, but they also die sooner than animals fed diets with carbohydrates.

Experts in the impact of nutrition on health across the animal kingdom, Professors Stephen Simpson and David Raubenheimer, note that a diet composition that sustains maximum reproductive output or leanness is not the same as that which best supports longevity. In other words, different diets might be useful for different purposes: reducing body weight and increasing reproductive capability versus living a longer life. Certainly, as I mentioned in Chapter 8, the consumption of whole grains is very consistently associated with health benefits and a reduction in the risk of early death. The traditional Mediterranean diet also has by far the strongest evidence base for health benefits, and this is a diet quite high in complex carbohydrates, such as wholegrain cereals and legumes.

Should we avoid legumes?

The short answer? No! Legumes are a key component of the Mediterranean diet and an important source of fibre. Extensive evidence from observational studies shows that eating more legumes is associated with a reduction in heart disease, blood pressure and cholesterol. The effect on cholesterol appears to be related to soluble fibre content, which binds to bile acids and decreases reabsorption. Bile acids are favoured by the inflammation-associated *Bilophila* bacteria in our guts, so this may be another way that legume consumption benefits health.

Legumes are rich in protein, slow-release carbohydrates, dietary fibre, micronutrients, and other bioactive components associated with health benefits. As well as epidemiological (observational) evidence, there's also experimental evidence for protective effects against chronic disease. They may also help with weight loss, as they increase the sense of fullness and satiety, and have a low glycemic load – meaning they release their energy slowly.

Some people have suggested that legumes should be avoided because they weren't part of our Paleolithic diets (we've already addressed this one) and because of their lectin content. Lectin is a type of protein that binds to carbohydrates, and is found in legumes, grains and some vegetables. It's commonly referred to as an 'anti-nutrient', as lectins are not digestible and can bind to the cells lining the digestive tract, which may disrupt nutrient absorption. Some individuals report symptoms such as bloating or gastrointestinal discomfort as a result of eating foods containing lectin, and thus exclude legumes from their diet.

While these negative effects seem worth avoiding, there's little scientific evidence suggesting that avoiding lectin-containing foods is a good idea for most people. Much of the research on the negative effects of lectins is based on early animal studies where lectins were consumed in high concentrations and in isolation in a controlled laboratory environment. These studies suggested that lectin consumption in animals was associated with disruptions to the health and function of the cells lining the gut wall, altered gut microbiota and immune function, increased inflammation and changes to the overall growth and health of the animals; however, these studies have not been replicated in humans.

Importantly, humans do not consume lectins in isolation. Lectins are consumed as part of whole foods, and the various preparation process of whole grains and legumes – soaking, fermenting and cooking – decrease the lectin content of these foods, mitigating any potentially problematic effects. This means that lectin-containing foods are quite okay when consumed as part of the human diet, and scientific evidence for the benefits of legumes and wholegrains far outweighs the concerns of trace amounts of lectins. Personally, these foods form the basis of many of my meals and I eat them several times a week.

Which fats are healthy?

There are few areas of nutrition science where there's more debate and misinformation on health benefits or otherwise than with dietary fats, especially saturated fats. In particular, diets that derive the majority of their energy intake from fats (such as the ketogenic diet) have become increasingly popular, and there is much debate about the traditional advice to avoid saturated fats for health. Recent meta-analyses have stirred up the saturated fat and heart disease controversy, but in the opinion of most nutrition experts, the best controlled intervention studies, and the best conducted meta-analyses still show that replacing saturated fat with mono- and polyunsaturated fats reduces the risk of cardiovascular disease. (For a useful recent review of the saturated fat–heart health issues, conducted as an 'Evidence Check' rapid review for the National Heart Foundation, refer to the executive summary or conclusion of P. Clifton and K. Keogh in the Sources.)

However, the importance of considering whole foods and dietary patterns rather than single nutrients cannot be overstated here. Whole foods with saturated fat come with vitamins, polyphenols and all sorts of protective factors, whereas processed foods do not. This includes processed meats, which have recently been linked to the serious psychiatric condition mania on the basis of their nitrate content. Related to this is what you are replacing the saturated fat with. If you replace it with food sources containing mono- or polyunsaturated fatty acids (from foods such as avocados, nuts, olives and fish), this is cardio-protective. But if you replace saturated fats with processed carbohydrates, which is what many people did on the basis of dietary recommendations, then saturated fat may be healthier in comparison. This concept is what many of the controversial meta-analyses missed. To give you a real-life example, a bit of full-fat Greek yoghurt or blue cheese is unlikely to promote heart disease, but a full-fat doughnut or sausage will!

We've also spoken in some detail about the evidence related to high-fat diets in animals, and saturated fats in relation to the gut microbiota, where they have been found to adversely affect the gut microbiome by reducing the good *Bifidobacteria* and increasing the pro-inflammatory *Bilophila* bacteria. Saturated fats are also linked to inflammation, and cognitive decline and dementia risk in most human studies, and to leaky gut and brain inflammation in animal studies. Thus, there is enough evidence there to suggest a negative impact of saturated fat consumption at high levels.

Personally, I love a bit of blue and stinky cheese and full-fat natural yoghurt in my diet, but I don't eat processed meats such as sausages and bacon.

There are two other key dietary fats that come under a lot of scrutiny and tend to come with a lot of misinformation attached: olive oil and coconut oil.

Olive oil

This is a very important source of monounsaturated fatty acids, although it needs to be the extra virgin type, not the more processed versions, to have the high levels of antioxidants that make it especially good for us. Extra virgin olive oil is the oil extracted from the first pressing of the olives. There's a myth that cooking with olive oil above a certain heat causes the production of toxic by-products. This may be true when cooking with oils that are primarily polyunsaturated fatty acids, which are not stable at high heats, such as soybean and canola oils, but it doesn't appear to be true for olive oil, which is primarily made up of monounsaturated fatty acids. These monounsaturated fats (as well as saturated fats) are actually quite stable at high heats.

As long as you're using the good stuff, the evidence from new scientific studies is that even when exposing olive oil to high heats for long periods of time, the quality and nutritional properties of the oil are largely unaffected. In real-world situations, you're unlikely to be using olive oil to cook for many hours at very high heats, meaning that it's even less likely that the health benefits of extra virgin olive oil are lost when it's used for cooking. The bottom line is that olive oil is a key element of the Mediterranean diet, with extensive evidence for its health benefits, and it should be the oil of choice for cooking. I love it and try to have two to three tablespoonfuls of it every day.

Coconut oil

This is the fat du jour. It seems to be in everything these days, particularly if you frequent trendy cafes and health-food stores. The popularity of coconut oil stems, I think, from some basic misunderstandings, and its overconsumption may be problematic, just as the overconsumption of saturated fats from animal sources is. The misunderstandings relate to a component of coconut oil called medium-chain triglyceride (MCT). MCT is a semi-synthetic laboratory product made up of two fatty acids called caprylic and capric acids. It was originally designed to be used in clinical settings for people who were malnourished but couldn't properly metabolise fat. There's some evidence that MTC aids in weight loss, although that tends to come with some rather nasty side effects, such as nausea and diarrhoea.

Because coconut oil has some naturally occurring caprylic and capric acids, its consumption has been proposed as a means of promoting weight loss. There is no empirical evidence for this idea, however, and coconut oil is primarily made up of lauric acid, which is a form of saturated fat. Scientific studies have found that coconut oil increases the production of LDL cholesterol (the type linked to heart disease) more than some vegetable oils, but slightly less so than butter. That said, it also seems to increase the 'good' HDL cholesterol. There is no scientific evidence behind the idea that coconut oil might kill pathogenic bacteria and viruses.

The bottom line? Consumed in small amounts as part of a varied diet, coconut oil is unlikely to do you any harm and it can be enjoyed for its flavour and versatility. But until there's scientific evidence showing particular health benefits (which there isn't as yet), you shouldn't be going out of your way to include it in your diet.

Do we especially need high-tryptophan foods?

Tryptophan is a precursor to the 'happy hormone' serotonin, so there's a widespread belief that consuming tryptophan or foods high in tryptophan, such as turkey or cottage cheese, might improve mood. There's no good evidence, however, that taking tryptophan as a supplement, or consuming foods high in tryptophan, has a benefit for mental health.

Tryptophan requires the use of a transport molecule to cross the blood–brain barrier for conversion to serotonin. Several other amino acids (tyrosine, phenylalanine, valine, leucine and isoleucine) compete to act as this transport molecule. Because almost every protein-containing food has other amino acids in it besides tryptophan, the presence of these competing amino acids restricts the transport of tryptophan into our brain. Indeed, even a tiny amount of protein in foods is enough to prevent an increase in tryptophan, and even high-carbohydrate foods typically still contain enough protein to have this effect. One very large study of nearly 30,000 people showed no association between the consumption of foods high in tryptophan and either mood or suicide.

Ironically maybe, it's actually high-carbohydrate foods that increase serotonin in the brain. When we eat a food high in carbohydrates, our body releases insulin, excessive levels of which cause tryptophan to move into the brain. Once in the brain, it triggers increased production of serotonin and melatonin, making you feel sleepy and relaxed. This is probably one reason why sweet foods seem to 'comfort' us. Interestingly, the gut microbiota play an important role in converting tryptophan into serotonin, so this is another factor to consider. Healthier guts might produce more serotonin via this mechanism.

There have been some double-blind, placebo-controlled studies of tryptophan as a supplement to improve mood, but the sample sizes were all quite small, and less than half of the studies showed statistically significant benefits of tryptophan supplements over a placebo. Importantly, there are many side-effects that can result from taking tryptophan supplements, including nausea, diarrhoea, drowsiness, lightheadedness, headache, dry mouth, blurred vision, and sedation. Even more importantly, tryptophan taken as a dietary supplement has the potential to cause serotonin syndrome (aka serotonin toxicity) when combined with other antidepressant drugs targeting the serotonergic system, such as SSRIs. This is quite serious. For all these reasons, I'd suggest that tryptophan supplements are probably *not* a good idea.

Is pyroluria a real health condition?

Again, no. Pyroluria is also known as pyrrole disorder, krypto-pyroluria, kryptopyrrole or mauve disorder. Those that consider this a true disease propose that pyroluria is an imbalance involving an abnormality in synthesis of haemoglobin (the oxygen-carrying molecule in blood), caused by genetic or environmental exposures such as 'toxins', stress or leaky gut. It is believed to result in the overproduction of pyrrole compounds that bind to zinc and vitamin B_6, leading to deficiencies in these vitamins and minerals that contribute to mental disorders. The proponents of pyroluria give a long list of symptoms that supposedly arise from this condition.

Many health practitioners and private labs offer kits or provide services that analyse the presence of pyrroles and related metabolites, and suggest treatment by supplementation with vitamin B_6, zinc and/or borage oil containing omega-6 fatty acids.

An avoidance of copper-containing foods and environmental sources of copper is also commonly recommended.

Where did this idea come from? An association between high levels of pyrroles in the urine of patients with a schizophrenia diagnosis was identified by one research group in the 1970s. Subsequently, a series of studies were conducted that failed to find the same results. Because of the lack of any evidence (indeed, there's much better evidence that it doesn't exist), there's been almost no research in this area in recent decades. We can therefore safely cross this one off our list of potential contributors to mental disorders. At the Food & Mood Centre, we don't think there's any reason to study this further; the existing evidence is strong enough to rule out pyroluria as a real health condition.

Key facts

- Some studies suggest that vegetarians have worse mental health than those who eat red meat, although we don't know if this is cause or effect, or the result of some third factor.
- We found that women eating either very little or a lot of red (unprocessed) meat were roughly twice as likely to have a clinical mood or anxiety disorder compared to those who ate the amount recommended in the Australian dietary guidelines, even when we took overall diet quality into account. Correlation or causation? We don't know.
- There's mixed evidence for an association between dairy foods and mental health, and intervention studies are needed to try to understand the possible impact of different types of dairy on mental health outcomes. Fermented dairy, such as kefir and yoghurt, are likely to provide health benefits.

- The premise of Palaeolithic diets is now outdated, with our new knowledge of the gut microbiota as our primary organ of adaptation.

- There's very little evidence, but not no evidence, for non-coeliac gluten sensitivity, but it seems that it is the FODMAP aspect of grains, rather than gluten itself, that promotes gut symptoms in some people.

- One small study suggests that gluten may prompt depressive symptoms in some people, but much more research is required to confirm this.

- Case and anecdotal reports suggest that some people with schizophrenia may have food sensitivities that can exacerbate their symptoms, but far more research is needed to confirm this.

- The evidence for the health benefits of wholegrain cereals and legumes is very extensive.

- Long-term low-carbohydrate diets are associated with poorer health outcomes and early death. Apparent short-term benefits may arise from weight loss rather than the removal of carbohydrates from the diet. Low carbohydrate diets reduce dietary fibre and have a negative impact on gut microbiota.

- The evidence against saturated fats, and for mono- and polyunsaturated fats, for health is very extensive. Consideration of the quality of the food in which these fats are found is, however, very important. Replacing saturated fats with highly processed vegetable oils or refined carbohydrates is highly problematic for health, and this may explain divergent research findings.

- Cooking with extra virgin olive oil does not lead to the production of toxic by-products, and extra virgin olive oil is an excellent source of polyphenols and monounsaturated fats.

- There's no evidence for particular health benefits of coconut oil. It's fine to use for flavour, but it's high in saturated fats and has been shown to increase 'bad' cholesterol as well as 'good' cholesterol.
- There's no good evidence for consuming 'tryptophan-rich' foods or tryptophan supplements for mental health.
- There's no evidence for, and quite a bit of evidence against, the existence of the condition 'pyroluria'.

12

The best diet for mental and brain health

Now that you've read everything in this book about the impact of diet and nutrition on the brain and the risk of mental and emotional disorders, I'm really hoping you're feeling motivated to take charge of your pantry. Just as importantly, I also hope you're inspired to make sure that the next generations do a lot better than we have! If you do feel this way, then read on.

You would have noticed a recurring theme throughout this book: the Mediterranean diet. The traditional Mediterranean diet is by far the dietary pattern with the largest and strongest research evidence base for health benefits, including mental health. A meta-analysis that included both observational and intervention data from nearly 13 million people showed that the Mediterranean diet reduced the risk of overall mortality, cardiovascular diseases, coronary heart disease, myocardial infarction, overall cancer incidence, neurodegenerative diseases and type 2 diabetes. And we know that it's clearly associated with a reduced risk of depression.

But that doesn't mean that the Mediterranean diet is the only dietary pattern that's healthy. Many other 'diets' have been associated with a reduced risk of depression, as well as other beneficial health outcomes. These include the 'dietary approaches to stop hypertension' (DASH) diet of fruit, vegetables, whole grains, healthy fats, lean red meats, fish, poultry and low-fat dairy; the traditional Norwegian (Nordic) diet of oily fish (salmon, mackerel and herring), whole grains (rye, oats and barley), vegetables (especially root vegetables and cruciferous vegetables such as cabbage, cauliflower and broccoli), wild and grass-fed meats, berries, yoghurts and kefir; the traditional Japanese diet of fresh and pickled vegetables, lots of fish, soy products (tofu and edamame beans), buckwheat and wholewheat noodles, and fermented foods (tempeh, miso, natto, seaweed and green tea); and traditional Anglo-Saxon diets of fruit, vegetables, unprocessed red meats, fish and whole grains.

Of course, these diets all have one overarching theme: whole, unprocessed foods, with an emphasis on plant foods, lean and unprocessed animal foods (fish and grass-fed red meats), healthy (unsaturated) fats from plant and fish (i.e. olive oil, oily fish and nuts), and wholegrain cereals.

Why are we so confused?

Unfortunately, as we've discussed, the media has provided an enormous amount of misinformation and debate about what comprises an ideal diet, much of it driven by the vested interest Big Food has in keeping us confused. But the biggest areas of debate have been around saturated fats and carbohydrates.

I won't go into huge detail as we covered this in the previous chapter, but it's important to clarify a few things here. First, the evidence from human and animal studies tells us that in the long term, diets low in complex carbohydrates and/or high in saturated fats, particularly animal fats, are linked to increased mortality (i.e. early death), and the risk of cardiovascular disease, cancer, type 2 diabetes and even cognitive decline (dementia). What the research tells us is that the most important factor affecting life span seems to be the balance (ratio) of carbohydrates to proteins. This understanding comes from our colleagues in Australia at the Charles Perkins Centre, Professors Simpson and Raubenheimer, who are regarded as the world experts in understanding the interactive effects of multiple nutrients on health, life span, ageing, and reproduction via what is called nutritional geometry. Based on very extensive research, nutritional geometry can define and quantify the consequences of different diet compositions on multiple measures of health across the animal kingdom – from insects to humans. What they have established is that across the animal world, diets with a high carbohydrate to protein ratio are consistently associated with increased life span and improved cardiometabolic outcomes.

If we apply this to humans, diets that are high in a diverse range of complex carbohydrates – from whole grains (e.g. brown rice, barley, rye, whole wheat, quinoa, whole oats, freekeh and buckwheat), starchy root vegetables (sweet potato, carrots, potato and pumpkin), fruit, and legumes (lentils, chickpeas and beans) – and relatively lower in protein (particularly from animals) are the ones we should aim for to increase our life span and reduce our risk of chronic disease. (As I noted before, a diet higher in protein and lower in carbohydrates seems to optimise leanness and reproduction, but at the expense of life span.) Indeed, such a diet is quite like the healthy peasant diet consumed widely in Britain during the mid-Victorian era, which I discussed at the start of the book. We'll have a closer look at what this healthy approach involves in real terms further on.

Are dietary guidelines helpful or harmful?

I think a lot of the confusion and debate regarding what to eat for good health has arisen from problems in the details and interpretation of the dietary guidelines that have been in place in many countries since the 1970s.

When the initial Dietary Goals for Americans proposed increasing carbohydrates and decreasing saturated fat and cholesterol in the diet, these recommendations stemmed at least partly from the belief that because levels of cholesterol in blood were linked to an increase in heart disease risk, foods high in cholesterol must increase the risk of heart disease. We now know, however, that the link between dietary cholesterol and our body's cholesterol levels aren't necessarily straightforward. For most people, the amount of cholesterol eaten has only a modest impact on the amount of cholesterol circulating in the blood, but in a small number of people, blood cholesterol levels rise and fall very strongly in relation to the amount of cholesterol eaten. For these 'responders', avoiding cholesterol-rich foods can have a substantial effect on blood cholesterol levels. This seems to be dependent on your genetic background.

The problem with the Dietary Goals for Americans was, however, not so much the recommendation to reduce saturated fats – given too much saturated fat does seem to be problematic for heart health, brain health and the composition of the gut microbiota – but that people (and food manufacturers) then replaced these fats with *refined* carbohydrates, such as processed cereals, and low-fat dairy foods with lots of added sugar. Just as importantly, the overall intake of calories went up due to increases in serving sizes, more foods eaten out of the home, and the increased availability of highly processed foods. So instead of reducing saturated fat and replacing it with healthy fats from olive oil, fish, nuts and avocados and complex carbohydrates from the sources I've just listed, they replaced their saturated fats with even more highly processed breakfast cereals; white or highly processed 'brown' breads, sweetened low-fat yoghurts and other low-fat foods; and a range of other non-complex carbohydrates; with a big fat serving of takeaway junk and processed foods on top. No wonder the population's blood sugar went up and everyone got fat and sick!

A large study from Harvard University, which included data from 52 countries, showed that raised blood glucose is responsible for 21 per cent of deaths from heart disease and 13 per cent of deaths from stroke worldwide. The authors noted that the impact of higher than optimal blood glucose levels is three times higher than of full-blown type 2 diabetes globally, because of the large number of people affected. We've already noted that high blood glucose (even high within the 'normal' range) is linked to dementia, and that high blood glucose during pregnancy may contribute to neurodevelopmental issues in children. The authors of this study noted that the consumption of any source of carbohydrate, over and above that from vegetables, fruit and whole grains, was harmful to human health. For me, this highlights that *possibly the most important aim for our long-term health is keeping our blood sugar low and stable by avoiding the intake of added sugars and refined carbohydrates.* But that doesn't mean avoiding carbohydrates altogether. It means avoiding *refined* carbohydrates, including added sugars, and consuming only complex carbohydrates from truly wholegrain cereals, legumes, fruits and vegetables.

These original dietary guidelines did recommend replacing saturated fats with plant fats, but they didn't specify that these should be the healthiest versions of plant oils – extra virgin olive oil and omega-3 fatty acids from seafood. Instead, people were told to replace butter and other cooking oils with margarines, which were (at the time) high in trans fats – extremely bad for health and now banned in many places – and omega-6 fatty acids from refined seed and vegetable oils, which oxidise easily and can be pro-inflammatory. Better to eat butter!

In many countries, we still have official dietary guidelines in place that are – in my opinion and that of many other health researchers – not ideal in that they don't specify in enough detail that carbohydrates need to be whole and unprocessed, and that fats and oils should come mainly from olive oil, avocados, oily fish and nuts. They also don't put enough emphasis on vegetables, fruit and legumes as important sources of carbohydrates. I really like the new (2015) healthy eating pyramid from Nutrition Australia, the bottom tier of which comprises these foods, with grains the second tier up (and with a bit more detail about what they actually mean by whole grains).

Similarly, the new recommendations based on plates are really useful for understanding what a main-meal plate should look like. This is pretty simple really: you should aim to fill half your plate with a diverse range of vegetables and/or salads, a quarter should have a good source of unprocessed protein (fish, unprocessed grass-fed red meat, tofu or another legume source of protein, ricotta or cottage cheese), and the final quarter a proper whole grain (brown rice, barley, quinoa, millet or similar). Then I'd add whole nuts, maybe some lovely ricotta or goat's cheese (if this wasn't already my main protein source), and a liberal dash of olive oil to really plump up the nutrition content.

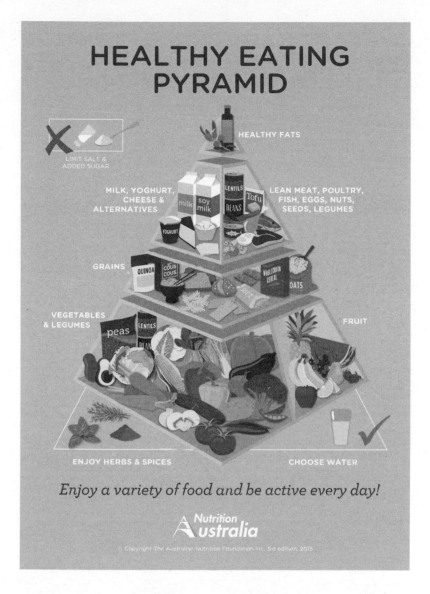

HEALTHY EATING PYRAMID

LIMIT SALT & ADDED SUGAR

HEALTHY FATS

MILK, YOGHURT, CHEESE & ALTERNATIVES

LEAN MEAT, POULTRY, FISH, EGGS, NUTS, SEEDS, LEGUMES

GRAINS

VEGETABLES & LEGUMES

FRUIT

ENJOY HERBS & SPICES

CHOOSE WATER

Enjoy a variety of food and be active every day!

Nutrition **Australia**

© Copyright The Australian Nutrition Foundation Inc. 3rd edition, 2015

The US-based 'MyPlate' is a bit confusing, with its recommendation that the vegetable/salad half of the plate could also include fruit – I'd personally save that for dessert! It also only specifies that half your grains should be whole grains.

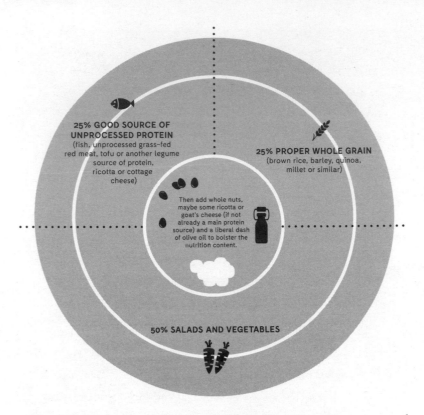

25% GOOD SOURCE OF UNPROCESSED PROTEIN
(fish, unprocessed grass-fed red meat, tofu or another legume source of protein, ricotta or cottage cheese)

25% PROPER WHOLE GRAIN
(brown rice, barley, quinoa, millet or similar)

Then add whole nuts, maybe some ricotta or goat's cheese (if not already a main protein source) and a liberal dash of olive oil to bolster the nutrition content.

50% SALADS AND VEGETABLES

But keeping it super-simple, I think the Brazilians have trumped everyone with their new dietary guidelines. These really boil down to: *Eat real food, mostly stuff that has grown in Brazil for centuries, with other people.* They also give great guidance on not just what to eat, but how to shop, cook and eat.

THE BRAZILIAN DIETARY GUIDELINES

- Make natural or minimally processed foods the basis of your diet.
- Use oils, fats, salt and sugar in small amounts when seasoning and cooking.
- Limit consumption of processed foods (they even include bread here, so maybe the bread in Brazil is not so great).

- Avoid consumption of ultra-processed foods (fatty, sweet or salty packaged snacks, biscuits, ice creams and confectionery in general; fizzy drinks and other soft drinks; sweetened juices and 'energy' drinks; sweetened breakfast cereals; cakes and cake mix, and cereal bars; sweetened and flavoured yoghurts and dairy drinks).
- Eat regularly and carefully in appropriate environments and, whenever possible, with other people.
- Avoid snacking between meals. Eat slowly and enjoy what you're eating, without engaging in another activity. Eat in clean, comfortable and quiet places, where there's no pressure to consume unlimited amounts of food. Whenever possible, eat in company, with family, friends, or colleagues.
- Shop in places that offer a variety of natural or minimally processed foods.
- Choose vegetables and fruits that are locally grown and in season. Whenever possible, buy organic and agroecological-based foods, preferably directly from the producers.
- Develop, exercise and share cooking skills, especially with boys and girls. If you don't have these skills – men as well as women – acquire them.
- Plan your time to make food and eating important in your life.
- Out of home, choose places that serve freshly made meals and avoid fast-food chains.
- Be wary of food advertising and marketing.

The SMILES study diet

Here is the diet we used in the SMILES study. As I mentioned earlier, this diet was developed using everything we knew to date about diet and mental health, and was based on both a traditional Mediterranean diet and the Australian dietary guidelines. Dr Rachelle Opie, our wonderful dietitian who developed the diet, called it the Mod*i*Med Diet to signify that it was a modified version of a traditional Mediterranean diet. It was specifically designed to be easy to make and follow, and inexpensive. Rachelle's top ten tips and Mod*i*Med diet pyramid, along with a sample meal plan and a sample recipe from the SMILES study, appear in the Appendix (page 293).

What I eat myself

I'm going to finish up now with a few dietary suggestions from my own home. As you might imagine, given my interest in food, I've always eaten a pretty healthy diet. Like many people, however, I've tended to eat more than I actually need (particularly because I love food so much). Also, being stupidly busy and a bit of a workaholic, I sometimes bolt my food or use it for energy when I'm tired, rather than eating only when I'm hungry. This has meant that over recent years (particularly as I hit menopause) I'd put on extra kilos and was no longer in the healthy weight range. In 2016 I was diagnosed out of the blue with breast cancer. I had to have major surgery, but luckily avoided chemotherapy or radiotherapy. My oncologist told me that I needed to lose weight to reduce the risk of getting it again, so I've worked hard to lose weight over the last two years (nothing like a life-threatening illness to prompt health changes). I now habitually eat less than I did before (and eat more slowly), while making sure I get all my key food groups (and lots of diversity – very important) each day. So what I suggest here takes quantity into account, as well as quality.

I'll start with a broad, simple understanding of some of my food basics, followed by some simple recipes.

Breakfast options in my home

Wholegrain, sourdough toast (one slice) with: avocado, hummus, tomato, goat's cheese, eggs or tomato, or a combination of these. You can even add Vegemite to your avocado toast. Or peanut butter (not the highly processed stuff with added sugar and salt, but the decent stuff), tahini or some other form of nut butter. Sardines or mackerel are also great options, as they will give you a terrific hit of protein and omega-3 fatty acids. Try to find the tinned sardines in olive oil.

'Breakfast mush': This is my favourite go-to brekky. I start with whatever non-starchy vegetables I have in the fridge – I want them water-based so that they cook quickly. I would usually include zucchini, mushrooms, leeks (if you have them – they're an excellent source of fibre), tomatoes, spinach and herbs from my garden – chopped quickly and roughly (the idea here is to do this quickly so you're not late for work). Put them all into a shallow pan with a lid, add some extra virgin olive oil and a splash of water, and cook for five minutes over a low heat until the vegies are soft. Then add eggs that have been mixed with a bit of milk. I mix all mine together into a bit of a slop, but you can keep the scramble separate if you like. I use roughly one and a half eggs per person. I then add more herbs, season with salt and pepper and serve in a bowl. My husband has his on a slice of wholegrain sourdough toast. Sometimes I add a bit of either ricotta or goat's cheese on top. To be honest, a version of this is often lunch or dinner as well! Too easy.

Porridge: *Not* the pre-cooked 'instant' kind, but whole oats (preferably steel-cut) that you can soak overnight if you like, or just cook slowly on the stove. I have mine with some milk or soy milk, plus some frozen berries. My husband likes to add currants and sultanas, or sliced fruit. Keep your serves small (half a cup uncooked). I really love oats. If I was stuck on a desert island for the rest of my life and could only have one food to take with me, it would be oats.

Muesli: *Not* the toasted kind (granola) that has been cooked in oil and has loads of sugar/honey added. You can make your own pretty easily, and include some nuts and seeds, as well as oats, spelt flakes, and so on. There are many recipes online. Again, you can eat this with fruit or added nuts and seeds. Keep your serves small (half a cup uncooked). I sometimes like to put mine in the fridge overnight, soaking in milk or soy milk, so that I can have it soft and cold with yoghurt and fruit in the morning.

Yoghurt: This is pretty simple. I take two tablespoons of whole plain yoghurt (I love Greek yoghurt), then sprinkle some muesli or oats on top and add a bit of frozen or fresh fruit.

Smoothie: I don't have this for breakfast very often, mainly because I find it doesn't give me enough 'bulk' to keep me full until lunchtime, but it's a great way to get yoghurt (or home-made kefir – even better) into your day. I use my own kefir if I have it (or yoghurt), a little bit of frozen banana, frozen blueberries and any sort of milk (cow's milk or soy or almond milk). You can put some oats in there as well if you like. You can get pretty creative and there are lots of recipes online.

Sunday fry-up: On the weekend, I'll sometimes do a bit of a traditional English extravaganza, with eggs, cooked mushrooms and tomatoes, avocado, baked beans, goat's cheese and sourdough bread. I use butter and really enjoy every mouthful! No bacon, though. Apart from the health impact of processed meats, the way pigs and other animals are treated in industrial agriculture is appalling. As I noted earlier, I'm largely vegetarian mainly for that reason.

Buckwheat pancakes: I love buckwheat and it's a healthy option for pancakes. It's high in fibre and minerals, as well as protein, so it keeps you full. I use plain buckwheat flour, pour water and milk and an egg into a well in the middle of the flour, then mix it all up to a runny consistency and cook it in a pan. Add sliced banana for extra yum.

My lunch options

I usually take my lunch to work with me or visit the little Lebanese café next door to work, where they do a fantastic falafel and a simply amazing silverbeet and lentil soup (with lemon) in winter.

Falafel: with hummus and salad. You can buy pre-made falafels (and pre-made vegetable/bean/lentil burgers) at the supermarket. Just add a good-quality hummus or make your own in a blender.

Homemade salad: with nuts and goat's or ricotta cheese, olive oil and balsamic vinegar. Sometimes I used tinned fish, such as salmon or tuna instead of the nuts. I try to get lots of different sorts of greens into my salads, such as lettuces, spinach leaves, radicchio and watercress, which I grow in pots outside my kitchen. I then add grated carrots (extra points if you can use the purple ones), grated (raw) beetroot, tomatoes, herbs and sometimes even some chopped cabbage instead of the dark-green leaves, just for a change.

Soup: I'm the master of the soup and make these very quickly at home. If you have a blender, they're super-easy. You can use tinned beans or other legumes. Cook onion, garlic and vegies with homemade stock or a stock cube, add the legumes, blitz them in the blender and you're good to go! I like cannellini beans and cauliflower, but you can really get creative here. There are a million good recipes online. You can bulk up your soups by adding barley, which is very cheap and delicious in soups. I also like to add parmesan cheese for flavour. You can make a big batch of soup on the weekend, then freeze it in portions to take to work for lunch. Easy.

Rye crackers with toppings: such as cottage or ricotta cheese, tinned fish, tomatoes, avocado or whatever you fancy (I'm a bit addicted to hummus). You can also use nut butters. This quick, easy and very tasty lunch is commonly eaten in Norway, where they add smoked salmon, which is delicious (but also expensive and very salty, so not for everyday use). I've been in Norway again recently and eaten their fantastic knekkerbrød, which is a sort of cracker made with whole grains and lots of seeds. I'm determined to learn to make it at home.

Baked or fried tempeh: I wouldn't have this on its own, but I do add it – chopped up – to salads, or eat it with avocado, brown rice and some sesame oil or a bit of soy sauce. Tempeh is made from fermented soybeans, so has the added goodness from the fermentation process, as well as being high in fibre and protein. It's a great substitute for meat, as it has that umami flavour and a similar texture.

Wholegrain sourdough with topping: Again, use whatever takes your fancy from the lists above. I like to drizzle it with olive oil before I come to work, then add whatever option I've brought with me (cottage or ricotta cheese, tinned fish, tomatoes, avocado, hummus, nut butter, and so on). I particularly love avocado with hummus, topped with sliced spring onions and a drizzle of soy sauce or tamari. Yum!

Left-overs: This one needs no explanation – whatever I've made for dinner the night before often ends up on my plate the next day for lunch.

My dinner options

For dinner, I make soups, wholegrain pasta or brown rice with various sauces based on vegetables, or simply steamed vegies with fish and brown rice (I like simple). I make a minestrone soup that keeps me going all week.

NO PACKAGED PROCESSED FOODS

One big thing you'll notice about my daily menus and food lists is the lack of foods that come in packages. The exception to that would be tinned fish and beans, and pre-cut salads, which I use a lot (this is my version of 'fast food'), and a few healthy but quick breakfast options. Something like 70 per cent of the world's biggest companies make processed foods. Essentially this means that they take the original ingredients, then change them. They add (usually bad) stuff, take (usually good) stuff away, and put it into a package to sell. If they didn't do this, there'd be nothing for them to sell and no way to make their massive profits. Can you see why they'd prefer people not to adopt my sort of diet?

Handy hints for a healthy home

(Sorry – I love a bit of alliteration and I'm easily amused.)

These are what are in and out in my home, but your list might be a bit different depending on your cultural background.

Pantry staples IN

Dried legumes: such as adzuki beans, kidney beans, white/haricot beans, black beans, black-eyed peas, lima beans, pinto beans, lentils (red, green, brown, du Puy), split peas, whole peas and chickpeas. All of these (apart from the red lentils) I soak in a bowl of water for a few hours before cooking. Stick them in the fridge before you leave for work in the morning.

Tinned legumes: such as borlotti beans, chickpeas, cannellini beans, red beans, three-bean mix, lentils

Tinned tomatoes

Tinned fish: tuna, salmon and sardines

Wholegrain cereals: whole oats (although quick-cook oats are okay for emergencies such as running late for work!), unsweetened muesli, barley, brown rice (red and wild rice are also nice, but more expensive), couscous, freekeh, millet, quinoa, polenta, farro

Pasta: I have buckwheat and wholemeal pasta, but good-quality durum wheat pasta is okay as well, particularly if you cook it and allow it to cool before reheating. This increases the resistant starch content and reduces the calories!

Wholewheat flour, spelt flour, buckwheat flour (stone-ground/minimally milled)

Spices: cumin, garam masala, bay leaves, chilli powder and flakes, cinnamon, cloves, coriander (ground and seeds), curry powder, fennel seeds, ground ginger, paprika, peppercorns, turmeric and sumac

Good-quality Australian extra virgin olive oil (lots!)

Balsamic and apple cider vinegar

Honey and maple syrup

Stock cubes

Dried porcini mushrooms or mushroom powder (this is expensive, but you don't need much and it really elevates vegetarian dishes to the next level)

Fried shallots (yum)

Sesame oil

Soy sauce or tamari

Rice wine vinegar
Mirin
Sweet chilli sauce

Pantry staples OUT

Processed breakfast cereals (even the ones that say 'low salt' or
'low sugar' or 'full of grains' are usually a no-no; even granola
is usually full of sugar and fat)

Snack foods such as potato chips, corn chips, pretzels, biscuits,
sweets, soft drinks and cordials (diet or sugar-sweetened)

Two-minute noodles, pre-packaged sauces (unless low-salt/sugar,
such as low-sodium pasta sauce), macaroni cheese, instant soups

Breakfast and most muesli bars, pancake mixes, cake mixes, tinned
rice desserts, condensed milk, fruit bars, muffins, waffles

White bread, 'high-fibre' white bread, any bread where white flour
is an ingredient (many brands will try to convince you of their
health properties, but check the label for white flour, sodium
levels and added emulsifiers and sugars). This includes bagels,
unfortunately

White flour (even if it says organic or unbleached, it's still low in
fibre and high in not much else that's good)

Fridge staples IN

Bearing in mind that I'm mainly vegetarian, so your fridge might
also include organic grass-fed red meat and organic chicken. I would
strongly suggest you avoid non-organic meat and chicken because
of the overuse of antibiotics in these animals. Antibiotics are used to
make farm animals fatter (and may do the same for us) as well as for
preventing and treating disease. Although there have been changes
in some countries recently to reduce the use of antibiotics in the
food chain, more than 70 per cent of antibiotics in the US are used

for farm animals. Antibiotic resistance is a very scary issue and – of course – they can wreak havoc on our gut microbiota.

Vegetables and fruit (three-quarters of my fridge, obviously)

Free-range eggs

Raw nuts and seeds: walnuts, almonds, cashews, brazil nuts, hazelnuts, pine nuts, pumpkin seeds, sunflower seeds, sesame seeds (I store all of these in the fridge to keep them fresh)

Tempeh, quark, tofu, natural and Greek yoghurt (I variously use cow's and sheep yoghurt, but also make my own kefir), ricotta or cottage cheese, and blue cheese and natural cheese, such as brie or cheddar (for treats)

Fresh fish and shellfish, such as oysters or mussels (not always, but regularly)

A big tub of hummus

Fermented veg of some sort (sauerkraut, for example, but not the pasteurised version)

Tahini, miso paste, peanut butter (not the ones with added salt and sugar)

Homemade vegetable stock (this isn't necessary, but it is nice!)

Milk (I use low-fat but full-fat is okay, as long as you're not having a huge amount every day)

Soy milk (made with whole soybeans, not isolates)

Butter (I love butter, but I use it sparingly as a treat)

Soda water (I have a machine for making my own)

Grapefruit juice or other non-sweetened fruit juice (I use this in small quantities like cordial, to mix with the soda water)

Fridge staples OUT

Processed meats: bacon, ham, turkey roll, chicken roll, hot dogs, sausages, salami, kabana, mortadella

Yoghurts and other dairy with added sugar or artificial sugars

Flavoured and sweetened rice desserts, or versions thereof

Processed cheese and cheese spreads

Soft drinks, with or without artificial sweeteners, and other drinks with added sweeteners (milk drinks, fruit juices and so on)

Freezer staples IN

Blueberries

Other berries

Edamame beans

Frozen vegetables of different types

Frozen prawns and marinara mix

Pre-packaged vegetable/bean burgers from the supermarket, for emergencies

Good-quality bread (I like to make my own, then slice it before freezing)

Freezer staples OUT

Ice cream and other ice desserts

Frozen fried products, such as nuggets, chips, pies, pastries, battered fish and meats

Frozen pizza or similar

*

I'll finish off with reinforcing an important caveat that I mentioned earlier: there are many ways to eat a healthy diet and I don't think it's useful to get militant about one style of diet over another. People respond to food in very individual ways that likely relate to their own microbiota fingerprint as well as their cultural backgrounds and beliefs about food. As long as what you're eating has a high amount and diversity of plant foods and is low in junk and processed foods, you'll be doing better than about 90 per cent of the population these days! Getting too hung up worrying about what to eat and what not to eat can be bad for your mental health, just like a junk food diet can be. One way of thinking about it that I find useful is, 'Don't eat anything your grandmother wouldn't recognise,' (within reason of course). Just learn to love vegetables and legumes, experiment with simple recipes, and try to eat like a peasant. This can be good for your wallet as well as your health.

Conclusion

The evidence from the study of the mid-Victorians highlights so clearly and beautifully just how profoundly our food supply and environment can affect population health. Our current food supply is broken, and governments currently lack the will or the power to change things. Until we – with our wallets and our votes – can get them to act, it's critical that we take things into our own hands.

Ultra-processed foods make up a large and increasing component of our daily diets, and their ubiquity, affordability and marketing means that we've increasingly replaced our traditional wholefood diets with eating patterns that are high in energy and damaging additives, and low in fibre and nutrients. While we've been told for years that this will mean more illness and early death from chronic diseases, only recently have we understood the implications for our mental health and the health of our brains throughout our lives.

Food and nutrition are fundamental to every aspect of our functioning. Using a car analogy, if we put dirty, watered-down petrol in, we're not going to get the performance or durability we want or expect. But until medical practitioners are trained to understand the importance of diet to mental and brain health, and until governments and policymakers recognise that they must put aside the pressure from Big Food and change our food environment, we must act ourselves.

It's incumbent on all of us to become warriors for the health of our family, friends and communities. We need to lead by example, not only by providing whole, nutritious food for our families, and teaching them to shop for, cook and enjoy real food, but also by bringing pressure on our local officials to improve the food environment in our own neighbourhoods. Schools, in particular, need to be a focus of change. Many local communities raise funds to create small vegetable gardens within schools, but such options are not the standard in many communities. Consider working with fellow parents to try to do something similar in your local schools. Also consider taking up options for cooking classes in your neighbourhood, or maybe even start a cooking club yourself. At the very least, learn the basics and pass these on to your children and grandchildren! Very importantly, learn to recognise when Big Food is manipulating your behaviour and food choices. Be critical in your evaluation of the messages you hear and the advertising you're exposed to, and teach your children to do the same. You don't want to pay the price of your and your family's health just so industry can increase its profits. Unfortunately, this is exactly what's been happening since the late 1800s. See it for what it is and call it out!

I'd like you to finish this book with a very clear message that what we put in our mouths really matters, both in the short and long term. Don't be seduced by the promise of fast, cheap, tasty food – the price you pay will *really* not be worth it.

PART 2
RECIPES FOR GOOD MENTAL HEALTH

Introduction

My formal education is in psychology and epidemiology, not nutrition, so everything I know about food comes from my research and my personal passion. I'm extremely lucky, however, to work with an amazing team, many of whom have many years of formal education in nutrition research. This team has been very helpful to me in writing this book and providing me with the most up-to-date and comprehensive research evidence concerning diet and nutrition.

Meg Hockey and Dr Tetyana Rocks (yes, that really is her name, and we're all very jealous) have designed these recipes, which focus on simple wholefood ingredients and meals that are inexpensive, easy to prepare and delicious. Meg is a PhD student with the Food & Mood Centre; I first met her when she was doing her undergraduate studies in nutrition and she came to work as an intern on the SMILES study. There's not a person in the world who could meet Meg and not be struck by her beautiful nature *and* her amazing talents and work ethic. Tetyana is also a joy. She came to us when we were interviewing for the Food & Mood Centre's first postdoctoral research fellow. She walked into the interview, sat down and announced that her two loves in life (apart from her daughters) were 'food and research'. They're my passions as well, so I fell completely in love with her. Now her highly infectious laugh and expansive personality mean that we all compete to make her lose her lunch (funny cat videos work really well, we've found). Tetyana is from the Ukraine, where their traditional diet includes many unique fermented foods. Recipes for some of these are included at the end of this section.

These Mediterranean-style recipes are quick, easy and cheap to make – and so tasty. Experiment with different vegetables and fruit to vary the flavours and depending on the season.

Breakfast

Banana bruschetta

Serves 1

100 g (1 small) banana
50 g blueberries or strawberries
80–100 g (2 slices) quality wholemeal or wholegrain bread
100 g ricotta cheese
20 g slivered almonds or other nuts of your choice, toasted in a
    dry frying pan
1 teaspoon honey, for drizzling

1. Thinly slice the banana and strawberries.
2. Toast the bread.
3. Spread ricotta on the toast and top with the sliced fruit.
4. Sprinkle with the nuts and drizzle with the honey. Serve.

Sweet and fruity quinoa

Serves 1

70 g quinoa
100 ml milk of your choice
100 g (1 small) banana, apple or pear
200 g strawberries
50 g blueberries
10 g slivered almonds
1 teaspoon honey
2 teaspoons lime, lemon or orange juice

1. Cook the quinoa according to package instructions using the milk mixed with the necessary quantity of water. Cool slightly.
2. Chop the banana and strawberries, if necessary, into bite-size pieces.
3. Gently mix the banana and strawberry into the quinoa.
4. Serve topped with the blueberries and almonds, and drizzled with the honey and juice.

Summer berry bowl

Serves 1

30 g rolled oats, or barley or buckwheat flakes
1 teaspoon honey, for drizzling
20 g mixed nuts and seeds of your choice (such as pecans, almonds, pumpkin seeds)
100 g (1 small) banana

200 g frozen mixed berries
150 g Greek yoghurt

1. Set aside 1 teaspoon each of the rolled oats or flakes, honey, and mixed nuts and seeds. Slice the banana and set half aside.
2. Process the remaining ingredients in a food processor or blender until smooth.
3. Transfer to a small bowl, top with the reserved flakes, banana, nuts and seeds, and drizzle with the reserved honey.

Bircher muesli

Serves 1

40 g oats
80 g apple or orange juice
10 g dried apricots
10 g almonds
10 g walnuts
10 g pumpkin seeds
3 teaspoons currants or sultanas
150 g plain or Greek yoghurt
100 g small apple, pear or any other fresh fruit of your choice
½ teaspoon cinnamon
1 teaspoon honey, for drizzling

1. Place oats in a medium bowl or screw-top jar and pour over the juice.
2. Chop the apricots, almonds and walnuts and add to the soaked oats.

3. Add the pumpkin seeds, currants and yoghurt, and mix well.
4. Cover the mixture and refrigerate for at least 2 hours or overnight.
5. Chop the apple.
6. Serve in a bowl, topped with the apple, sprinkled with the cinnamon and drizzled with the honey.

Fruity pancakes

Serves 1

1 large egg
80 ml cow's milk or kefir
2 teaspoons extra virgin olive oil
30 g almond meal
150 g apple
50 g blueberries
1 teaspoon honey

1. Whisk the egg, then continue whisking while gradually adding the milk or kefir, oil and almond meal.
2. Grate the apple and add to the mixture with half the blueberries.
3. Heat a dry non-stick frying pan over medium heat. Cook the pancakes one at a time until lightly golden on both sides, turning once.
4. Serve topped with the remaining blueberries and a drizzle of honey.

Tomato and avocado bruschetta

Serves 1

150 g (1 large) Roma tomato
100 g avocado
100 g (2 slices) heavy bread (such as rye, spelt)
60 g ricotta or cottage cheese
10 g fresh herbs (such as basil, coriander, parsley, chives)
salt and black pepper, to taste
2 teaspoons dukkah (optional)

1. Thinly slice the tomato and mash the avocado.
2. Toast the bread and spread with the ricotta while still hot.
3. Top with the mashed avocado, sliced tomato and fresh herbs, then season with salt, pepper and dukkah (if using). Serve immediately.

Lunch

Open Mediterranean sandwich

Serves 1

50 g red onion
50 g red capsicum
50 g zucchini
50 g pumpkin
2 teaspoons extra virgin olive oil
salt and dried rosemary, to taste
60 g (1 large) slice wholemeal sourdough bread
1 tablespoon hummus
2 teaspoons balsamic vinegar
2 teaspoons dukkah, or crushed nuts of your choice
feta and fresh herbs, to serve (optional)

1. Preheat the oven to 200°C.
2. Slice the onion, capsicum and zucchini. Peel and slice the pumpkin.
3. Arrange the sliced vegetables in a medium roasting tin. Drizzle with the balsamic vinegar, olive oil and sprinkle with salt and rosemary.
4. Bake for 15 minutes, adding the bread to the oven for the last 2–3 minutes to toast it.
5. Spread the bread with the hummus, top with the baked vegetables and sprinkle with the dukkah. Crumble over the feta and scatter with fresh herbs (if using).

Tip: You can easily make hummus at home. Drain and rinse 400 g tinned chickpeas. Blend them in a food processor or blender with 1 tablespoon lemon juice, 2 tablespoons extra virgin olive oil and 1 tablespoon boiling water. Season with a pinch each of salt and black pepper.

Moroccan chickpea salad

Serves 1

150 g carrot
20 g red onion
10 g coriander leaves
150 g tinned chickpeas, drained and rinsed
3 teaspoons currants
50 g cooked couscous
1 teaspoon Moroccan spices

Dressing

2 teaspoons extra virgin olive oil

2 teaspoons lemon juice

1. Peel and grate the carrot, slice the onion and chop the coriander.
2. Combine all the ingredients in a medium bowl.
3. To make the dressing, mix the olive oil and lemon juice.
4. Toss the dressing through the salad and serve immediately.

Fresh salad with freekeh

Serves 2

200 g roma tomatoes

100 g lebanese cucumber

100 g yellow capsicum

50 g red onion

200 g avocado

20 g fresh herbs (such as basil, parsley, chives, coriander)

50 g mixed rocket and baby spinach leaves

150 g cooked freekeh

1 tablespoon fresh lemon juice

1 tablespoon extra virgin olive oil

20 g dry-roasted nuts (such as walnuts, almonds, hazelnuts), chopped

1. Slice the tomatoes, cucumber, capsicum, onion and avocado. Chop the herbs.
2. Place the rocket and spinach mix in a large bowl, then top with the freekeh, vegetables and herbs.
3. To serve, dress the salad with the lemon juice and olive oil, and sprinkle with the nuts.

Salad wrap

70 g cooked or tinned chickpeas
100 g avocado
2 teaspoons extra virgin olive oil
60 g tomato
20 g red onion
70 g (1 large) wholemeal wrap or flatbread
3 handfuls rocket
20 g feta
black pepper, to taste

1. Mash the chickpeas and avocado together with a fork and mix in the oil. Thinly slice or chop the tomato and onion.
2. Lay the wrap on a flat surface, then top with the rocket and mashed chickpeas and avocado. Add the tomato and onion and crumble over the feta.
3. Season with pepper, then wrap and serve.

Lunch lamb pita for one

Serves 1

90 g lamb steak, trimmed
2 teaspoons extra virgin olive oil
100 g zucchini
50 g (½ small) Lebanese cucumber
50 g cherry tomatoes

10 g Kalamata olives
40 g red onion
10 g mint
70 g (1 large) wholemeal pita bread
1 handful rocket
1 tablespoon Greek yoghurt
20 g feta cheese
salt and black pepper, to taste

1. Put your grill pan (stove) or BBQ grill on high.
2. Drizzle the lamb with half the olive oil and grill until just cooked. Set aside to rest for 2–3 minutes, then slice thinly.
3. Slice the zucchini lengthwise. Grill for 2–3 minutes, until soft and lightly browned.
4. Dice the cucumber, halve the tomatoes and olives, and chop the onion and mint.
5. Warm the pita bread according to the packet instructions.
6. Fill the pita with the lamb, zucchini, rocket, cucumber, tomato, onion, olives and mint. Drizzle with the remaining olive oil, top with a dollop of yoghurt and crumble over the feta. Season to taste and serve.

Dinner

Roast vegetables and barley salad

Serves 2

100 g pumpkin

100 g red capsicum

100 g baby carrots

100 g button mushrooms

100 g red onion

100 g baby squash

extra virgin olive oil, for drizzling

1 teaspoon cumin seeds

1 teaspoon fennel seeds

120 g pearl barley

100 g grapes

40 g cashews, toasted in a dry frying pan (or you can pop them in
    the microwave on a piece of paper towelling for 1 minute)

1 small handful herbs (such as basil, mint, parsley, coriander)

1 handful baby salad leaves

30–40 g cheese (such as blue cheese, goat's cheese)

Dressing

1½ tablespoons plain or Greek yoghurt

1 tablespoon extra virgin olive oil

1 tablespoon lemon juice

1 teaspoon garam masala or Middle Eastern spice mix

salt and black pepper, to taste

1. Preheat the oven to 220°C.
2. Peel the pumpkin. Cut the pumpkin and capsicum into 2 cm chunks. Halve the carrots and mushrooms lengthways. Cut the onion and squash into segments.
3. Lay the vegetables in a roasting tin, drizzle with olive oil and scatter with the cumin and fennel seeds. Bake for 30–40 minutes, until tender.
4. Bring 500–750 ml salted water to the boil in a large saucepan. Add the barley and cook for 25–30 minutes or until tender. Drain and keep warm.
5. Meanwhile, halve each grape lengthways. Chop the nuts and herbs.
6. To make the dressing, whisk all of the ingredients together in a small bowl.
7. Spread the salad leaves on a large platter. Top with the cooked barley, baked vegetables, grapes, nuts and herbs. Drizzle with the dressing and serve.

Spicy salad with farro, brussels sprouts and chickpea crisps

Serves 2

240 g tinned chickpeas, drained and rinsed

extra virgin olive oil, for drizzling

2 teaspoons cumin seeds

2 teaspoons fennel seeds

120 g farro

300 g brussels sprouts

1½ tablespoons currants

Dressing
1 tablespoon extra virgin olive oil

1½ tablespoons lemon juice

2 teaspoons lemon zest

1 garlic clove, finely chopped

pinch of chilli flakes

salt, to taste

1. Preheat the oven to 200°C and line a baking tray with baking paper.
2. Spread the chickpeas on the prepared baking tray. Drizzle with olive oil and scatter with the cumin and fennel seeds. Roast for 30 minutes or until golden and crispy.
3. Meanwhile, cook the farro according to the packet instructions. Keep warm.
4. Cut the brussels sprouts into segments. Bring 1 litre water to the boil in a large saucepan. Blanch in the boiling water for 1 minute then drain and toss with the farro and currants.

5. Transfer the farro mixture to a large serving bowl, then top with the chickpeas.
6. To make the dressing, combine all the ingredients in a small bowl.
7. Toss the dressing through the salad and serve warm.

Lentil soup with barley and vegetables

Serves 2

100 g brown onion
1 garlic clove
50 g celery
200 g red capsicum
1 tablespoon extra virgin olive oil
2 teaspoons fennel seeds
100 g (½ cup) red lentils
50 g (¼ cup) pearl barley
400 g tinned diced tomatoes
400 ml low-salt vegetable stock
1 tablespoon lemon zest
1 tablespoon lemon juice
20 g parsley, finely chopped
salt, to taste
2 tablespoons Greek yoghurt
80 g (2 slices) wholemeal sourdough bread, toasted

1. Finely chop the onion, garlic, celery and capsicum.
2. Heat the olive oil over medium–low heat in a medium heavy-based saucepan. Add the fennel seeds and cook for 1–2 minutes, until fragrant.
3. Add the onion, garlic and celery and sweat for 2–4 minutes.

4. Stir in the lentils and barley and cook for 3–4 minutes.
5. Add the tomatoes and capsicum and cook, stirring gently, for 2–3 minutes.
6. Add the stock, increase the heat to medium–high and bring to the boil, then reduce the heat to low and simmer, covered, for 40–50 minutes, until the barley and lentils are soft.
7. Add the lemon zest and juice and the parsley. Season with salt.
8. Serve the soup with a dollop of yoghurt on top and toast on the side.

Mediterranean bowl

Serves 2

100 g tri-colour quinoa
lemon slices, to serve (optional)
feta, ricotta or cottage cheese, to serve (optional)

Marinated tofu
120 g firm tofu
2 teaspoons extra virgin olive oil
1 tablespoon lemon juice
1 teaspoon dried oregano

Bowl fillers
50 g broccoli
100 g cherry tomatoes
200 g avocado
100 g Lebanese cucumber
50 g red cabbage
50 g snow peas

50 g zucchini

40 g red onion

50 g kale

1 small handful parsley leaves

20 g black or Kalamata olives, sliced

20 g slivered almonds

Dressing

2 tablespoons plain or Greek yoghurt

1 tablespoon extra virgin olive oil

1 tablespoon lemon juice

2 teaspoons balsamic or apple cider vinegar

salt and black pepper, to taste

1. To marinate the tofu, cut the tofu into 1 cm dice. Drizzle with the olive oil and lemon juice, then scatter with the oregano. Cover and set aside to marinate for at least 30 minutes.
2. Cook the quinoa according to the packet instructions. Keep warm.
3. Boil, microwave or steam the broccoli until just cooked.
4. Cut each tomato into halves or quarters, depending on their size. Chop the avocado and cucumber into 1 cm dice. Finely shred the cabbage and snow peas, and grate the zucchini. Thinly slice the onion and finely chop the kale and parsley.
5. To make the dressing, whisk all the ingredients together in a small bowl.
6. Fill two medium bowls in layers or wedges with quinoa, marinated tofu and vegetables.
7. Top each bowl with parsley, olives and almonds. Add lemon slices and cheese (if using). Drizzle with the dressing and serve.

Tip: Experiment with different combinations of vegetables, herbs and nuts to find your signature bowl.

Pasta with mushrooms and goat's cheese

Serves 2

100 g wholemeal pasta
500 g button mushrooms
2 garlic cloves
1 tablespoon extra virgin olive oil
2 teaspoons lemon zest
2 teaspoons lemon juice
1 teaspoon dried thyme
1 teaspoon dried rosemary
pinch or two of salt
2 handfuls rocket
40–50 g soft goat's cheese

1. Cook the pasta according to the packet instructions and keep warm.
2. Meanwhile, chop the mushrooms and finely chop the garlic.
3. Heat the olive oil in a large non-stick frying pan over medium heat. Add the mushrooms and fry gently until slightly golden.
4. Add the lemon zest and juice, garlic, thyme and rosemary, stirring gently. Season with salt and cook for a further 1–2 minutes.
5. Add the pasta and rocket and stir gently to combine. Cook until the pasta is warmed through and the rocket is slightly wilted.
6. Serve topped with the goat's cheese.

Smoky casserole

Serves 2

300 g eggplant
salt, for sprinkling
100 g brown onion
1 garlic clove
1 tablespoon extra virgin olive oil
1 teaspoon coriander seeds
1 teaspoon cumin seeds
1 teaspoon fennel seeds
pinch of smoked paprika
240 g tinned chickpeas, drained and rinsed
300 g ripe tomatoes, roughly chopped
50 g feta or 2 tablespoons Greek yoghurt
80 g (2 small) wholemeal pita bread

1. Cut the eggplant into 2 cm dice. Transfer to a colander, sprinkle with salt and set aside to drain for 10–15 minutes.
2. Meanwhile, chop the onion and garlic.
3. Heat the olive oil in a large heavy-based saucepan over medium heat. Add the coriander, cumin and fennel seeds and cook for 3–4 minutes, until fragrant. Add the paprika and stir gently.
4. Add the onion and garlic. Reduce the heat to low and sweat for 3–5 minutes, until the onion is transparent.
5. Add the eggplant and cook, stirring occasionally, for about 10 minutes.
6. Add the chickpeas and tomatoes, then increase the heat to medium and bring to the boil. Reduce the heat to low, then simmer, covered, for 10 minutes.

7. Serve topped with crumbled feta or a dollop of Greek yoghurt and a pita bread on the side.

Warm barley with roast pumpkin, tofu and egg

Serves 2

2 large eggs
100 g firm tofu
100 g (½ cup) pearl barley
200 g pumpkin
2 tablespoons extra virgin olive oil
60 g baby spinach
20 g Kalamata olives
20 g soft goat's cheese
1 tablespoon lemon juice
salt and black pepper, to taste

Marinade
1 garlic clove, finely chopped
1 tablespoon lemon juice
1 tablespoon extra virgin olive oil
1 teaspoon ground cumin
1 teaspoon dried oregano

1. Preheat the oven to 200°C.
2. Hard-boil the eggs, then cool, peel and halve lengthways.
3. To make the marinade, combine all the ingredients in a small jar and shake well.

4. Cut the tofu into six slices and lay them in a shallow dish. Pour over the marinade, then cover and refrigerate for at least 20 minutes.
5. Meanwhile, cook the barley according to the packet instructions
6. Cut the pumpkin into 2 cm dice. Spread in a roasting tin and drizzle with half the olive oil. Bake for 10–15 minutes, until just cooked. Set aside to cool slightly.
7. Preheat a barbecue grill or non-stick chargrill pan to hot. Drain the tofu, retaining the marinade, and cook on each side for 3–5 minutes, until grill marks appear.
8. In a large shallow bowl, gently mix the spinach and barley. Arrange the eggs, tofu, pumpkin, olives and cheese on top. Drizzle with the reserved marinade, the remaining olive oil and the lemon juice. Season with salt and pepper and serve warm.

Eggplant pasta with mushrooms and nuts

Serves 2

200 g mushrooms
400 g (1 large) eggplant
200 g cherry tomatoes
200 g tinned diced tomatoes
1 tablespoon reduced-salt tomato paste
1 tablespoon white wine vinegar
1 teaspoon sugar
1½ tablespoons extra virgin olive oil
80 g wholemeal penne pasta
salt and black pepper, to taste

1 tablespoon capers, rinsed and drained
30 g pine nuts
30 g feta
1 small handful parsley leaves, chopped

1. Clean the mushrooms and slice lengthways. Cut the eggplant into 1 cm dice and halve each cherry tomato lengthways.
2. In a medium bowl, combine the tinned tomatoes, tomato paste, vinegar and sugar, mixing well.
3. Heat the olive oil in a large saucepan over medium heat. Add the eggplant, mushrooms and cherry tomatoes, and cook for 2–3 minutes.
4. Add the tinned tomato mixture and stir to coat the vegetables.
5. Reduce the heat to low and simmer, covered, stirring occasionally, for 20–25 minutes.
6. Meanwhile, cook the pasta according to the packet instructions.
7. Remove the lid from the eggplant mixture and cook for a final 3–5 minutes to thicken. Season with salt and pepper.
8. Drain the pasta and add to the eggplant sauce.
9. Serve topped with the capers, pine nuts, crumbled feta and parsley.

Cabbage and bean soup

Serves 2

100 g brown onion
2 garlic cloves
100 g potato

200 g cabbage

1 tablespoon extra virgin olive oil

2 teaspoons smoked paprika

2 teaspoons mixed dried herbs

400 g tinned diced tomatoes

240 g tinned cannellini beans, rinsed and drained

salt and black pepper, to taste

80 g (2 slices) wholemeal sourdough bread

2 tablespoons Greek yoghurt

1 tablespoon grated parmesan

1. Finely chop the onion and garlic. Peel and chop the potato. Shred the cabbage and massage with your fingers.
2. Heat the olive oil in a medium saucepan over low heat. Add the onion and garlic and cook for 1–2 minutes, until the onion is translucent.
3. Add the paprika and dried herbs, and cook for 3–4 minutes.
4. Add the potato and cook for a further 3–4 minutes.
5. Add the cabbage and cook for 2–3 minutes, until it begins to wilt.
6. Stir in the tomatoes and beans, and cook for 2–3 minutes.
7. Add enough water to completely cover the vegetables, then increase the heat to medium and bring to the boil. Reduce the heat to low and simmer, covered, for 10–12 minutes, until the potato is cooked.
8. Season with salt and pepper and serve with a slice of bread, a dollop of yoghurt and a scattering of parmesan.

Cannellini soup with kale and couscous

Serves 2

2 garlic cloves
200 g kale
1 tablespoon extra virgin olive oil
2 teaspoons allspice
salt and white pepper, to taste
300 g reduced-salt vegetable stock
240 g tinned cannellini beans, rinsed and drained
3 tablespoons wholemeal couscous
80 g (2 slices) wholemeal sourdough bread, to serve
fresh herbs, to serve

1. Finely chop the garlic and kale.
2. Heat the olive oil in a medium saucepan over low heat. Add the garlic and kale, season with the allspice, salt and pepper, and cook for about 5 minutes.
3. Add the stock and beans. Increase the heat to medium and bring to the boil, then add the couscous. Reduce the heat to low and simmer, covered, for about 10 minutes, until the couscous is cooked.
4. Serve with the bread on the side and herbs on top.

Grilled prawns with greens and white bean purée

Serves 2

150 g asparagus
100 g green beans or broccolini
250 g raw prawns, shelled and deveined
1 small handful parsley leaves, chopped
lemon wedges, to serve

White bean purée
360 g tinned cannellini beans, rinsed and drained
1 tablespoon extra virgin olive oil
1 garlic clove
pinch of salt

Dressing
1 tablespoon sherry or white wine vinegar
1 tablespoon lemon juice
3 teaspoons extra virgin olive oil
1 teaspoon caster sugar
pinch of saffron threads

1. To make the white bean purée, pulse all the ingredients in a food processor until smooth.
2. Blanch the asparagus and green beans in boiling water for 1 minute.
3. To make the dressing, whisk all the ingredients together in a jug.

4. Preheat a barbecue grill or non-stick chargrill pan to medium–high. Grill the prawns for 1–2 minutes on each side, until just cooked. Remove to a small bowl and cover with the dressing.
5. Spoon the purée onto a large platter, and top with the asparagus, beans and prawns. Garnish with parsley and serve with lemon wedges.

Italian-style salmon with couscous salad

Serves 1

1 garlic clove
40 g baby squash
40 g zucchini
80 g tomato
20 g spring onion
120 g salmon fillet, skin removed
pinch of paprika
pinch each of salt and black pepper
pinch of dried thyme
1 tablespoon lemon juice
lemon slices, to serve (optional)

Salad
30 g pearl couscous
1 small handful flat-leaf parsley
1 small handful spinach leaves
100 g Lebanese cucumber
20 g feta
1½ tablespoons currants

2 teaspoons extra virgin olive oil

2 teaspoons lemon juice

1 tablespoon Greek yoghurt

1. Preheat the oven to 200°C. Cut a 25 cm square of aluminium foil.
2. Thinly slice or finely chop the garlic. Slice the squash, zucchini, tomato and spring onion.
3. Lay the fish on the prepared foil and top with the vegetables. Sprinkle with paprika, salt and pepper. Scatter with the thyme and drizzle with the lemon juice.
4. Wrap the fish in the foil and bake for 15–18 minutes, until cooked through.
5. Meanwhile, make the salad. Cook the couscous according to the packet instructions.
6. Roughly chop the parsley and spinach, slice the cucumber and crumble the feta.
7. In a salad bowl, combine the couscous, cucumber, parsley, spinach, feta and currants and toss well. Dress with the olive oil, lemon juice and yoghurt and toss through.
8. Serve the fish with the vegetables and salad, topped with sliced lemon (if using).

Moroccan fish stew

Serves 2

70 g brown onion

1 garlic clove

1 cm piece of ginger

240 g firm white fish fillets, skin removed
1 tablespoon extra virgin olive oil
1 teaspoon ground cumin
1 teaspoon ground turmeric
pinch of cayenne pepper
good pinch of salt
200 g tinned diced tomatoes
200 g low-salt fish stock
120 g tinned chickpeas, drained and rinsed
70 g wholemeal couscous
1 handful coriander leaves, chopped
2 tablespoons Greek or plain yoghurt or light sour cream

1. Thinly slice the onion. Finely chop the garlic and ginger. Cut the fish into small chunks.
2. Heat the olive oil in a large heavy-based saucepan over medium heat. Add the onion, garlic and ginger, and cook for about 3–5 minutes, until the onion is translucent.
3. Add the cumin, turmeric, cayenne pepper, salt, tomatoes and stock. Bring to the boil, and simmer for about 5 minutes.
4. Add the fish and cook for a further 5 minutes.
5. Stir in the chickpeas and couscous. Simmer for 2 minutes, then remove from the heat, stir again and stand for 3–5 minutes.
6. Serve the stew topped with the coriander and a dollop of yoghurt.

Salmon patties

Serves 2

1 medium or half a large sweet potato
200 g zucchini
1 small handful fresh herbs (such as dill, chives)
180 g tinned salmon, drained
1 large egg, lightly beaten
50 g frozen peas
20 g spring onion, thinly sliced
2 tablespoons wholemeal flour
pinch each of salt and black pepper
1 tablespoon extra virgin olive oil
2 handfuls rocket
2 tablespoons Greek yoghurt
lemon wedges, to serve

1. Steam, microwave or boil the sweet potato until cooked.
2. Meanwhile, grate the zucchini. Chop the herbs, setting aside 2 tablespoons as a garnish.
3. Mash the sweet potato and combine in a large bowl with the salmon, egg, zucchini, peas, spring onion, herbs and flour. Season with the salt and pepper.
4. Divide the salmon mixture into eight portions and shape into flat patties.
5. Heat half the olive oil in a large non-stick frying pan over medium heat, and cook half the patties for 3–4 minutes on each side until golden. Repeat with the remaining oil and patties.
6. Serve the patties with a handful of rocket, a dollop of yoghurt, a lemon wedge for squeezing and a scattering of the reserved herbs.

Tip: These patties are excellent served in a (healthy) burger bun. Divide the mixture into two, shape into large patties and cook for 5–7 minutes on each side. Serve in a wholegrain sourdough bun with fresh salad vegetables of your choice.

Seafood penne

Serves 2

100 g red onion

2 garlic cloves

1 small red chilli or pinch of dried chilli

1 small handful parsley

100 g (2 cups) spinach leaves

1 tablespoon extra virgin olive oil

200 g seafood marinara mix

400 g tinned diced tomatoes

salt and black pepper, to taste

80 g wholemeal penne pasta

150 g frozen peas

1 tablespoon grated parmesan

1. Chop the onion, garlic, chilli and parsley. Wash and drain the spinach and set aside.
2. Heat half the olive oil in a medium non-stick frying pan over medium heat. Add the seafood mix and cook until tender.
3. Stir in the parsley, then remove to a bowl and set aside.
4. Return the frying pan to the heat and add the remaining olive oil. Add the onion and cook for 3–4 minutes, until translucent.
5. Add the garlic and chilli, and cook, stirring, for 2 minutes.

6. Add the tomatoes and cook until heated through. Season with salt and pepper.
7. Cook the pasta according to the packet instructions, adding the peas in the last 2 minutes of cooking. Drain, then add the spinach and stir through.
8. Serve the pasta topped with the sauce, seafood and parmesan.

Seafood paella with colourful vegetables

Serves 2

100 g (½ cup) brown rice
300 ml low-salt fish stock
100 g brown onion
1 garlic clove
100 g cherry tomatoes
50 g yellow, red or green capsicum
40 g black olives
1 tablespoon extra virgin olive oil
1 teaspoon smoked paprika
½ teaspoon cayenne pepper
pinch of saffron threads
pinch of salt
200 g seafood marinara mix
50 g (⅓ cup) frozen peas
50 g (⅓ cup) frozen corn
50 g frozen beans
1 small handful parsley and coriander leaves, chopped
lemon wedges, to serve (optional)

1. Combine the rice and fish stock in a medium saucepan over medium heat and bring to the boil. Reduce the heat to low and simmer, covered, for 25 minutes. Set aside with the lid on. Do not drain.
2. Meanwhile, chop the onion and finely chop the garlic. Halve the tomatoes and chop the capsicum and olives.
3. Heat the olive oil in a medium heavy-based saucepan over medium heat. Add the onion and garlic and cook, stirring, for 5 minutes, until the onion is translucent.
4. Add the spices, salt, seafood mix, peas, corn and beans, then cook for 5 minutes.
5. Add the tomatoes, capsicum, olives and rice, then reduce the heat to low and simmer for 5–10 minutes.
6. Serve topped with the parsley and coriander, with lemon wedges on the side (if using).

One-pan chicken with mushrooms, vegies and broad beans

Serves 1

50 g leek

1 garlic clove

150 g button mushrooms

50 g fresh or frozen broccoli

90 g skinless chicken breast fillets

1 tablespoon extra virgin olive oil

1 teaspoon dried thyme or a few thyme sprigs, leaves picked

1 tablespoon white wine vinegar

100 ml low-salt chicken stock
pinch each of salt and black pepper
100 g (2/3 cup) frozen broad beans
120 g cooked brown rice

1. Thinly slice the leek, garlic and mushrooms. If using fresh broccoli, cut into florets. Slice the chicken.
2. Heat the oil in a medium saucepan over medium–low heat. Add the leek and garlic and sweat for 2–3 minutes. Add the thyme and continue to sweat until the onion and leek are translucent.
3. Add the chicken and cook for 5 minutes.
4. Add the mushrooms, vinegar and chicken stock, and season with salt and pepper. Bring to the boil, then reduce the heat and simmer, covered, for 15 minutes.
5. Add the broad beans and broccoli, then cook for a further 2–3 minutes, or until cooked to your liking.
6. Serve with the brown rice.

Beef and vegetables soup

Serves 2

100 g brown onion
100 g carrot
100 g sweet potato
100 g potato
80 g celery
2 teaspoons extra virgin olive oil
140 g lean minced beef

2 teaspoons dried thyme

good pinch of salt

50 g (1/3 cup) frozen peas

50 g (1/3 cup) frozen corn

100 g frozen green beans

1–2 dried bay leaves

400 g tinned whole Roma tomatoes

black pepper, to taste

80 g (2 slices) wholemeal sourdough bread

2 tablespoons Greek yoghurt

1. Cut the onion, carrot, sweet potato, potato and celery into 1 cm dice.
2. Heat the olive oil in a large heavy-based saucepan over medium heat. Add the beef, thyme and salt, and cook for about 5 minutes, breaking up the mince as you cook.
3. Add the onion, carrot, sweet potato, potato and celery, then reduce the heat to low and cook for 5 minutes.
4. Add the peas, corn, beans, bay leaves, tomatoes and pepper. Depending on desired thickness, add 125–250 ml water. Increase the heat to medium and bring to the boil, then reduce heat to low and simmer, covered, for 20–30 minutes, until the vegetables are cooked.
5. Serve with fresh or toasted bread on the side and a dollop of yoghurt on top.

Summer roast salad

Serves 2

a few rosemary sprigs, leaves picked
200 g baby beetroot
olive oil, for drizzling
200 g baby new potatoes
120 g (2 small) red onions
150 g beef eye fillet
pinch each of salt, black pepper and mixed dried herbs
200 g baby green beans
20 g snow peas
100 g watercress

Dressing
1½ tablespoons balsamic vinegar
1 tablespoon extra virgin olive oil
2 teaspoons wholegrain mustard
1 teaspoon honey

1. Preheat the oven to 180°C.
2. Chop the rosemary. Wash the beetroot well and cut into quarters.
3. Spread the beetroot in a roasting tin, drizzle with olive oil scatter with half the rosemary.
4. Bake the beetroot on the bottom shelf for about 50 minutes, until cooked through.
5. Meanwhile, boil, steam or microwave the potatoes until just cooked. Cool slightly then cut into quarters. Peel the onions and cut into quarters.
6. Spread the potato and onion in a second roasting tin, drizzle with olive oil and scatter with the remaining rosemary.

7. Bake the potato on the middle shelf for about 20 minutes, until crisp and golden.
8. Meanwhile, heat a large non-stick frying pan over medium–high heat and cook the beef for 1–2 minutes on each side to seal.
9. Transfer the beef to an ovenproof dish, drizzle with olive oil and season with salt, pepper and mixed herbs. Bake on the top shelf for about 10 minutes. Remove from the oven and set aside to rest for 5 minutes, then slice thinly.
10. Bring some water to the boil in a medium saucepan and blanch the beans for about 1 minute. Drain.
11. Thinly slice the snow peas and mix with the watercress.
12. To make the dressing, whisk all the ingredients together in a small bowl.
13. Spread the watercress and snow pea mix on a large platter, then add the beans, beetroot, potato and onion. Top with the beef and drizzle with the dressing.

Lamb and barley with vegetables and feta pesto

Serves 2

120 g beetroot

120 g pumpkin

2 teaspoons extra virgin olive oil, plus extra as needed

2 teaspoons cumin seeds

1 teaspoon mixed spice

100 g (½ cup) pearl barley

150 g lamb steak, trimmed

1 tablespoon Greek yoghurt to serve

Feta pesto

1 tablespoon extra virgin olive oil
1 small handful mint leaves
1 small handful parsley leaves
1 garlic clove
40 g feta

1. Preheat the oven to 180°C.
2. Cut the beetroot into wedges and the pumpkin into 3 cm chunks. Spread in separate roasting tins.
3. Drizzle the vegetables with the olive oil and scatter with the cumin seeds and mixed spice. Bake the beetroot for about 15 minutes, then add the pumpkin and bake for a further 35 minutes or until cooked through, checking halfway.
4. Cook the barley according to the packet instructions. Keep warm.
5. To make the pesto, pulse the oil, mint, parsley and garlic in a small food processor until finely chopped. Crumble the cheese and stir into the pesto without processing further.
6. Heat a drizzle of olive oil in a large non-stick frying pan over medium heat. Cook the lamb for 2–3 minutes on each side or to your liking. Remove from the pan and rest for 1–2 minutes, then cut into thick slices.
7. Place the barley in a large serving bowl and top with the baked vegetables. Add the lamb and dress with the pesto and yoghurt to serve.

Fermented corner

Here are a couple of the best-loved traditional fermented dishes from Ukraine. Each uses simple common ingredients and is easy to prepare. For some of them you'll need a kitchen thermometer.

Important note: Please take care with kitchen hygiene. Keep your equipment and surfaces clean and sterilise your jars before you begin by running them through your dishwasher on a hot cycle. After all, we only want good bugs in our food!

Kisloe moloko (quick kefir)

This slightly fermented milk-based drink could be served on its own or used as a base for a cold soup (see recipe below) or a dressing in salads. Use it to make very fluffy pancakes or mix with fruit and nuts for a sweet dessert.

900 ml milk
100 g plain yoghurt or 100 ml kisloe moloko
1 teaspoon sugar

1. Pour the milk into a large saucepan, then warm over low heat to 35–40°C. (This will create an ideal environment for good bacteria to grow in your milk.) Cool the milk slightly.
2. Mix in the yoghurt and sugar. (The yoghurt will provide the starting bacterial cultures, while the sugar provides a little extra food for them to feast on.)
3. Transfer the mixture to a sterilised 1 litre glass jar and cover with a clean tea towel. (The idea is to have some air movement around the mixture while protecting it from the elements and invasion from foreign bugs.)
4. Keep the mixture at the room temperature (about 24°C) for 5–6 hours, then transfer to the fridge for a further 10–12 hours. Your kisloe moloko should be ready to enjoy, but it could take a touch longer, depending on your climate.
5. If you enjoy the taste, keep 100 ml as your new starter. Or you could experiment with a different yoghurt as your starter culture.

Ryazhenka

Ryazhenka is similar to kisloe moloko but is made from baked milk and has a slightly milder flavour. It's great to consume on its own or use in desserts.

1.5 litres milk
100 g plain yoghurt or 100 ml kefir
1 teaspoon sugar

1. Preheat the oven to 90–100°C.
2. Pour the milk into a large saucepan, then bring to the boil over low heat.
3. Transfer to an ovenproof dish, then bake for 4–5 hours. The milk will reduce in volume, darken in colour and form a caramel crust on top.
4. Cool the baked milk to 35–40°C and follow steps 2–4 of the kisloe moloko recipe.

Beetroot and greens soup with kefir

This is a great summer dish: easy to prepare, cool and fresh.

Serves 2

200 g beetroot
2 large eggs
200 g Lebanese cucumber
10 g spring onions
10 g chives
10 g dill
10 g basil leaves
10 g parsley leaves
10 g coriander leaves
50 g (1¼ cups) mixed green salad leaves
200 g Kisloe Moloko (page 285)
100 ml mineral water
salt and black pepper, to taste

1. Wash the beetroot well and place in a medium saucepan. Cover well with water and bring to the boil over medium heat.

Reduce the heat to low and simmer for 40–50 minutes or until soft. Cool, peel and cut into 5 mm dice.
2. Hard-boil the eggs. Cool, peel and cut into 5 mm dice.
3. Cut the cucumbers into 5 mm dice. Chop the spring onions, herbs and salad leaves.
4. Mix the kisloe moloko with the mineral water.
5. Combine the beetroot, cucumber, egg and greens in a large bowl and toss gently. Poor over the kefir mixture and toss again. Season with salt and pepper and serve immediately.

Kvashenaya kapusta (Ukrainian-style sauerkraut)

Kvashenaya kapusta is one of the staples of Ukrainian cuisine. It uses common vegetables, is easy to make and keeps well in the fridge. This is a basic recipe but you can add many other ingredients to enhance the flavour. For example, you could try serving it with herbs such as chives and spring onions or dill and dill seeds; sliced apple and onion; diced cooked potato; or even cooked meat.

To make kvashenaya kapusta, you'll need a 2.5 litre glass jar and a clean round rock that will fit into your jar and has about the same diameter. To clean your rock, boil it in water for 15–20 minutes.

2 kg cabbage
400 g carrots
40 g salt
2 teaspoons sugar
cooled boiled water, as needed

1. Wash and dry the cabbage and carrots, then finely shred both and transfer to a large bowl.
2. Mix the cabbage and carrot, then massage them thoroughly with your hands, until the vegetables soften and start to give up their juices.
3. Add the salt and sugar, and mix well.
4. Pack the cabbage and carrot into a sterilised jar as tightly as possible – keep pushing the vegetables down.
5. Pour the juices left in the bowl over the vegetables. If not completely covered, add cooled boiled water until just covered.
6. Top the jar with your clean rock to keep the vegetables in the juices and protect them from spoiling.
7. Keep at room temperature for 3–4 days or until little bubbles start to appear, then move to the fridge.
8. Serve your kvashenaya kapusta on its own or drizzled with a good olive oil.

Acknowledgements

Firstly, of course, I want to thank my family and friends from the bottom of my heart. It can't be easy loving a workaholic and I feel so grateful for the love and support you all give me, despite my regular absences, frequently furrowed brow and harassed demeanour!

I also want to acknowledge and profoundly thank Professor Michael Berk, who took me on as a work experience student when I was an undergraduate, and who has provided me with mentorship, sponsorship and friendship in the more than 15 years since. We make a great team Michael, and it continues to be a pleasure working with you. My thanks also go to my many wonderful mentors over the years: Professors Tony Jorm, Arnstein Mykletun, Jane Gunn and Kaarin Anstey. You have all been so generous in your support and time and I have learned so much from each of you.

I also want to thank my wonderful team at the Food & Mood Centre, many of whom helped me with sections of the book (particularly Chapter 11). You make coming to work a joy and

I'm so grateful to be able to work with you all to advance the field of Nutritional Psychiatry.

An enormous thank you also goes to both the Wilson Foundation and the Fernwood Foundation. So much of what we do would not be possible without the help of philanthropic donors like these and I am so grateful to the marvellous Karen Wilson and Di Williams for their partnership in our important endeavours.

Finally, a profound thank you to all the many members of the public who give up their time (and bodily samples!) to contribute to medical research. So much of what we know now is due to your efforts and involvement, even though you may not benefit personally from the research. I encourage everyone to participate in medical research so that future generations can have longer, healthier lives.

Appendix

The Modi Med Diet

ModiMed Diet top ten tips

1. Select fruits, vegetables and nuts as a snack.
   Eat 3 serves of fruit and 30 g (1½ tablespoons) unsalted nuts every day.

2. Include vegetables with every meal.
   Eat leafy greens and tomatoes every day.

3. Select wholegrain breads and cereals.
   Base your serving sizes on your activity levels.

4. Eat legumes three or four times a week.

5. Eat oily fish at least twice a week.

6. Eat lean red meat three or four times a week.
   Limit your serving sizes to 65–100 g.

7. Include two to three serves of dairy every day.
   Select reduced-fat products and plain yoghurt.

8. Use olive oil as your main added fat.
   Use 3 tablespoons extra virgin olive oil every day.

9. Save sweets only for special occasions.

10. Water is the best drink.

Sample Mod*i*Med Diet weekly meal plan

At first glance this plan may seem quite restrictive, but the idea was merely to provide guidance to the sorts of meals our participants could enjoy. It wasn't intended to be rigorously adhered to, with measuring, weighing and recording of food. During the study, recipes were provided for many of these options, along with salad and omelette ideas. A sample recipe plan is provided in this section.

Meal	Day 1	Day 2	Day 3
Breakfast	1 poached egg on 2 slices soy and linseed bread with avocado, tomato and spinach	2/3 cup wholegrain breakfast cereal with 1 tablespoon LSA and 250 ml reduced-fat milk	½ cup baked beans on 2 slices wholegrain toast with tomato, mushrooms, avocado and herbs
Morning snack	200 g Greek yoghurt with 1 cup fresh or frozen berries	An apple	An orange
Lunch	1–2 wholegrain flat breads with 95 g tinned tuna and green salad	Omelette with tomato, mushrooms and 20 g grated reduced-fat cheese, on 1–2 slices wholegrain toast	3 wholegrain crackers with salad and 20 g reduced-fat cheese
Afternoon snack	30 g almonds and 30 g dried fruit	An orange	An apple
Dinner	**Option 1** Grilled lamb steak with vegetables and brown rice **Option 2** Lamb casserole with brown rice	Lentil and vegetable soup with 20 g reduced-fat cheese and 2 slices wholegrain bread	Chicken pasta with vegetables and pesto
Supper	**Fruit smoothie:** 250 ml reduced-fat milk with a banana and 1–2 teaspoons honey	30 g almonds and 2 mandarins	2 kiwi fruit

Day 4	Day 5	Day 6	Day 7
30 g wholegrain breakfast cereal with 1 tablespoon LSA and 250 ml reduced-fat milk plus 1 cup berries	½ cup porridge with 250 ml reduced-fat milk and a banana	Omelette made with 1 egg, with red onion, tomato, herbs and 40 g grated reduced-fat cheese on 2 slices wholegrain toast	½ cup muesli with 1 tablespoon LSA, 30 g dried fruit, 125 ml reduced-fat milk and 100 g plain yoghurt
200 g Greek yoghurt with 2 teaspoons honey	100 g plain yoghurt with 30 g mixed nuts and 2 teaspoons honey	2 mandarins	30 g mixed nuts
1 poached omega-3 egg on 1 slice wholegrain bread with quinoa salad	2 salmon patties with feta, spinach and sweet potato salad	½ cup tinned four-bean mix with 1 cup salad vegetables and ½–1 cup couscous	**Option 1** Lamb patties with tzatziki and salad **Option 2** Spaghetti bolognese with salad
A banana	An apple	An orange and 15 g walnuts	2 kiwi fruit
Grilled salmon with broccoli, chilli and noodles and a salad	**Option 1** Honey and soy chicken stir-fry with brown rice **Option 2** Chicken casserole	Teriyaki beef stir-fry with cashews and noodles	½ cup baked beans with tomato, capsicum and mushrooms on 2 slices wholegrain bread
5 dates and 30 g almonds	2 kiwi fruit and 3 wholegrain crackers with 20 g reduced-fat cheese	200 g plain yoghurt with 1 cup berries	An apple

Sample meal plan recipe from the ModiMed Diet

Teriyaki beef stir-fry with cashews and noodles

Serves 4

400 g lean beef, cut into thin strips
2 garlic cloves, finely chopped
125 ml teriyaki marinade
400 g hokkien noodles
1½ tablespoons extra virgin olive oil
4 spring onions, cut into 5 cm lengths
250 g asparagus, trimmed, chopped
100 g snow peas, trimmed
200 g baby bok choy, quartered lengthways
200 g broccolini, halved lengthways
1 carrot, sliced
100 g unsalted cashew nuts

1. Place the steak in a bowl. Add the garlic and half the teriyaki marinade. Stir to coat. Cover and refrigerate for 30 minutes.
2. Place the noodles in a large, heatproof bowl. Cover with boiling water. Stand for 2 minutes. Drain. Separate the noodles.
3. Heat 1 tablespoon of the oil in a wok over high heat. Add the beef. Stir-fry for 2–3 minutes, until sealed. Remove to a plate.

4. Add the spring onions, asparagus, snow peas, bok choy, broccolini, carrot and remaining oil to the wok. Stir-fry for 1–2 minutes, until the asparagus is just tender. Return the beef and juices to the wok. Add the noodles, cashews and remaining teriyaki marinade. Stir-fry for 2 minutes or until heated through. Serve.

For a convenient alternative
1. Replace the noodles with instant rice.
2. Replace the fresh vegetables with frozen vegetables.

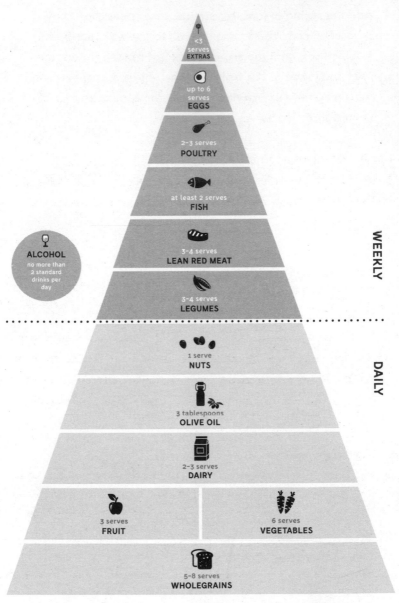

<3 serves
EXTRAS

up to 6 serves
EGGS

2–3 serves
POULTRY

at least 2 serves
FISH

3–4 serves
LEAN RED MEAT

3–4 serves
LEGUMES

1 serve
NUTS

3 tablespoons
OLIVE OIL

2–3 serves
DAIRY

3 serves
FRUIT

6 serves
VEGETABLES

5–8 serves
WHOLEGRAINS

WEEKLY

DAILY

ALCOHOL
no more than
2 standard
drinks per
day

Get daily exercise and enjoy meals with others

Drink plenty of water

The Mod*i*Med Diet food pyramid

Sources

I have consulted many more than 200 different scientific studies in writing this book but including all of them would have been unwieldy. As such, I've tried to provide the key references, favouring systematic reviews and meta-analyses where they are available.

*

Akbaraly, T. N., et al. (2009). 'Dietary pattern and depressive symptoms in middle age.' *Br J Psychiatry* **195**(5): 408–13.

Anhe, F. F., et al. (2015). 'A polyphenol-rich cranberry extract protects from diet-induced obesity, insulin resistance and intestinal inflammation in association with increased Akkermansia spp. population in the gut microbiota of mice.' *Gut* **64**(6): 872–83.

Attuquayefio, T. and R. J. Stevenson (2015). 'A systematic review of longer-term dietary interventions on human cognitive function: Emerging patterns and future directions.' *Appetite* **95**: 554–70.

Beilharz, J. E., et al. (2015). 'Diet-Induced Cognitive Deficits: The Role of Fat and Sugar, Potential Mechanisms and Nutritional Interventions.' *Nutrients* **7**(8): 6719-6738.

Berk, M., et al. (2013). 'So depression is an inflammatory disease, but where does the inflammation come from?' *BMC Medicine* **11**: 200.

Biesiekierski, J. R., et al. (2011). 'Gluten causes gastrointestinal symptoms in subjects without celiac disease: a double-blind randomized placebo-controlled trial.' *Am J Gastroenterol* **106**(3): 508–14.

Biesiekierski, J. R., et al. (2013). 'No effects of gluten in patients with self-reported non-celiac gluten sensitivity after dietary reduction of fermentable, poorly absorbed, short-chain carbohydrates.' *Gastroenterology* **145**(2): 320–8.

Bilbo, S. D. and V. Tsang (2010). 'Enduring consequences of maternal obesity for brain inflammation and behavior of offspring.' *FASEB J* **24**(6): 2104–15.

Borge, T. C., et al. (2017). 'The importance of maternal diet quality during pregnancy on cognitive and behavioural outcomes in children: a systematic review and meta-analysis.' *BMJ Open* **7**(9): e016777.

Brietzke, E., et al. (2018). 'Gluten related illnesses and severe mental disorders: a comprehensive review.' *Neurosci Biobehav Rev* **84**: 368–75.

Chassaing, B., et al. (2015). 'Dietary emulsifiers impact the mouse gut microbiota promoting colitis and metabolic syndrome.' *Nature* **519**(7541): 92–6.

Chatterton, M. L., et al. (2018). 'Economic evaluation of a dietary intervention for adults with major depression (the 'SMILES' trial).' *BMC Public Health* **18**(1): 599.

Cherbuin, N., et al. (2012). 'Higher normal fasting plasma glucose is associated with hippocampal atrophy: The PATH Study.' *Neurology* **79**(10): 1019–26.

Christ, A., et al. (2018). 'Western Diet Triggers NLRP3-Dependent Innate Immune Reprogramming.' *Cell* **172**(1-2): 162–75 e114.

Clayton, P. and J. Rowbotham (2009). 'How the mid-Victorians worked, ate and died.' *Int J Environ Res Public Health* **6**(3): 1235–53.

Clifton, P. and J. Keogh. Dietary fats and cardiovascular disease: an Evidence Check rapid review brokered by the Sax Institute for the National Heart Foundation of Australia, 2017, https://www.heartfoundation.org.au.

Croll, P. H., et al. (2018). 'Better diet quality relates to larger brain tissue volumes: The Rotterdam Study.' *Neurology* **90**(24): e2166–73.

Curtis, J., et al. (2016). 'Evaluating an individualized lifestyle and life skills intervention to prevent antipsychotic-induced weight gain in first-episode psychosis.' *Early Interv Psychiatry* **10**(3): 267–76.

Desrosiers, T. A., et al. (2018). 'Low carbohydrate diets may increase risk of neural tube defects.' *Birth Defects Res* **110**(11): 901–09.

Devkota, S., et al. (2012). 'Dietary-fat-induced taurocholic acid promotes pathobiont expansion and colitis in Il10-/- mice.' *Nature* **487**(7405): 104–8.

Dipnall, J. F., et al. (2015). 'The association between dietary patterns, diabetes and depression.' *J Affect Disord* **174**: 215–24.

Duncan, S. H., et al. (2007). 'Reduced dietary intake of carbohydrates by obese subjects results in decreased concentrations of butyrate and butyrate-producing bacteria in feces.' *Appl Environ Microbiol* **73**(4): 1073–8.

Eskelinen, M. H., et al. (2008). 'Fat intake at midlife and cognitive impairment later in life: a population-based CAIDE study.' *Int J Geriatr Psychiatry* **23**(7): 741–7.

Estruch, R., et al. (2013). 'Primary prevention of cardiovascular disease with a Mediterranean diet.' *N Engl J Med* **368**(14): 1279–90.

Fardet, A. and Y. Boirie (2014). 'Associations between food and beverage groups and major diet-related chronic diseases: an exhaustive review of pooled/meta-analyses and systematic reviews.' *Nutr Rev* **72**(12): 741–62.

Francis, H. and R. Stevenson (2013). 'The longer-term impacts of Western diet on human cognition and the brain.' *Appetite* **63**: 119–28.

Food and Agriculture Organization of the United Nations (2006). 'Food-based dietary guidelines – Brazil', revised edition 2014, http://www.fao.org.

Fung, T. T., et al. (2010). 'Low-carbohydrate diets and all-cause and cause-specific mortality: two cohort studies.' *Ann Intern Med* **153**(5): 289–98.

Gardner, C. D., et al. (2018). 'Effect of Low-Fat vs Low-Carbohydrate Diet on 12-Month Weight Loss in Overweight Adults and the Association With Genotype Pattern or Insulin Secretion: The DIETFITS Randomized Clinical Trial.' *JAMA* **319**(7): 667–79.

GBD 2016 Risk Factors Collaborators (2017). 'Global, regional, and national incidence, prevalence, and years lived with disability for 328 diseases and injuries for 195 countries, 1990-2016: a systematic analysis for the Global Burden of Disease Study 2016.' *Lancet* **390**(10100): 1211–59.

Haast, R. A. and A. J. Kiliaan (2015). 'Impact of fatty acids on brain circulation, structure and function.' *Prostaglandins Leukot Essent Fatty Acids* **92**: 3–14.

Hakkarainen, R., et al. (2003). 'Association of dietary amino acids with low mood.' *Depress Anxiety* **18**(2): 89–94.

Hiscock, H., et al. (2018). 'Paediatric mental and physical health presentations to emergency departments, Victoria, 2008-15.' *Med J Aust* **208**(8): 343–8.

Jacka, F., et al. (2010). 'Association of Western and traditional diets with depression and anxiety in women.' *The American Journal Of Psychiatry* **167**(3): 305–11.

Jacka, F. N., et al. (2009). 'Association between magnesium intake and depression and anxiety in community-dwelling adults: the Hordaland Health Study.' *Aust N Z J Psychiatry* **43**(1): 45–52.

Jacka, F. N., et al. (2010). 'Associations between diet quality and depressed mood in adolescents: results from the Australian Healthy Neighbourhoods Study.' *Aust N Z J Psychiatry* **44**(5): 435–42.

Jacka, F. N., et al. (2011). 'The association between habitual diet quality and the common mental disorders in community-dwelling adults: the Hordaland Health study.' *Psychosom Med* **73**(6): 483–90.

Jacka, F. N., et al. (2011). 'A prospective study of diet quality and mental health in adolescents.' *PLoS One* **6**(9): e24805.

Jacka F. N., et al. (2012). 'Red Meat Consumption and Mood and Anxiety Disorders.' *Psychother Psychosom* **81**: 196–8.

Jacka, F. N., et al. (2013). 'Maternal and early postnatal nutrition and mental health of offspring by age 5 years: a prospective cohort study.' *J Am Acad Child Adolesc Psychiatry* **52**(10): 1038–47.

Jacka, F. N., et al. (2015). 'Does reverse causality explain the relationship between diet and depression?' *J Affect Disord* **175**: 248–50.

Jacka, F. N., et al. (2015). 'Western diet is associated with a smaller hippocampus: a longitudinal investigation.' *BMC Med* **13**: 215.

Jacka, F. N., et al. (2017). 'A randomised controlled trial of dietary improvement for adults with major depression (the 'SMILES' trial).' *BMC Med* **15**(1): 23.

Kanoski, S. E. and T. L. Davidson (2011). 'Western diet consumption and cognitive impairment: links to hippocampal dysfunction and obesity.' *Physiol Behav* **103**(1): 59–68.

Kastorini, C. M., et al. (2011). 'The effect of Mediterranean diet on metabolic syndrome and its components: a meta-analysis of 50 studies and 534,906 individuals.' *J Am Coll Cardiol* **57**(11): 1299–313.

Kessler, R. C., et al. (2005). 'Lifetime prevalence and age-of-onset distributions of DSM-IV disorders in the National Comorbidity Survey Replication.' *Arch Gen Psychiatry* **62**(6): 593–602.

Khalid, S., et al. (2016). 'Is there an association between diet and depression in children and adolescents? A systematic review.' *Br J Nutr* **116**(12): 2097–108.

Khambadkone, S. G., et al. (2018). 'Nitrated meat products are associated with mania in humans and altered behavior and brain gene expression in rats.' *Mol Psychiatry*.

Krakowiak, P., et al. (2012). 'Maternal metabolic conditions and risk for autism and other neurodevelopmental disorders.' *Pediatrics* **129**(5): e1121–8.

Lachance, L. R. and K. McKenzie (2014). 'Biomarkers of gluten sensitivity in patients with non-affective psychosis: a meta-analysis.' *Schizophr Res* **152**(2-3): 521–7.

Lam, Y. Y., et al. (2015). 'Effects of dietary fat profile on gut permeability and microbiota and their relationships with metabolic changes in mice.' *Obesity (Silver Spring)* **23**(7): 1429–39.

Lassale, C., et al. (2018). 'Healthy dietary indices and risk of depressive outcomes: a systematic review and meta-analysis of observational studies.' *Mol Psychiatry*.

Laugesen, M. and R. Elliott (2003). 'Ischaemic heart disease, Type 1 diabetes, and cow milk A1 beta-casein.' *N Z Med J* 116(1168): U295.

Li, Y., et al. (2017). 'Dietary patterns and depression risk: A meta-analysis.' *Psychiatry Res* 253: 373–82.

Lucas, M., et al. (2013). 'Inflammatory dietary pattern and risk of depression among women.' *Brain, Behavior, and Immunity*.

Luppino, F. S., et al. (2010). 'Overweight, obesity, and depression: a systematic review and meta-analysis of longitudinal studies.' *Arch Gen Psychiatry* 67(3): 220–9.

Mari-Bauset, S., et al. (2014). 'Evidence of the gluten-free and casein-free diet in autism spectrum disorders: a systematic review.' *J Child Neurol* 29(12): 1718–27.

Martinez-Lacoba, R., et al. (2018). 'Mediterranean diet and health outcomes. a systematic meta-review.' *Eur J Public Health*.

McCann, D., et al. (2007). 'Food additives and hyperactive behaviour in 3-year-old and 8/9-year-old children in the community: a randomised, double-blinded, placebo-controlled trial.' *Lancet* 370(9598).

Miyazaki C., et al. (2015). 'Allergies in Children with Autism Spectrum Disorder: a Systematic Review and Meta-analysis.' *Rev J Autism Dev Disord* 2: 374.

Morris, M. C., et al. (2003). 'Dietary fats and the risk of incident Alzheimer disease.' *Arch Neurol* 60(2): 194–200.

Nanri, A., et al. (2013). 'Dietary patterns and suicide in Japanese adults: the Japan Public Health Center based Prospective Study.' *Br J Psychiatry* 203: 422–7.

Noto, H., et al. (2013). 'Low-carbohydrate diets and all-cause mortality: a systematic review and meta-analysis of observational studies.' *PLoS One* 8(1): e55030.

Novella, S. (2012). 'Pyroluria and Orthomolecular Psychiatry.' Science-Based Medicine, https://sciencebasedmedicine.org/pyroluria-and-orthomolecular-psychiatry/

O'Dea, J. A. (2003). 'Differences in overweight and obesity among Australian schoolchildren of low and middle/high socioeconomic status.' *Med J Aust* 179(1): 63.

Opie, R., et al. (2015). 'Assessing Healthy Diet Affordability in a Cohort with Major Depressive Disorder.' *Journal of Public Health and Epidemiology* 7(5): 159–69.

Parletta, N., et al. (2017). 'A Mediterranean-style dietary intervention supplemented with fish oil improves diet quality and mental health in people with depression: A randomized controlled trial (HELFIMED).' *Nutr Neurosci*: 1–14.

Pasco, J. A., et al. (2010). 'Association of high-sensitivity C-reactive protein with de novo major depression.' *Br J Psychiatry* 197: 372–7.

Pasco, J. A., et al. (2015). 'Milk consumption and the risk for incident major depressive disorder.' *Psychother Psychosom* 84(6): 384–6.

Peters, S. L., et al. (2014). 'Randomised clinical trial: gluten may cause depression in subjects with non-coeliac gluten sensitivity – an exploratory clinical study.' *Aliment Pharmacol Ther* 39(10): 1104–12.

Pina-Camacho, L., et al. (2015). 'Maternal depression symptoms, unhealthy diet and child emotional-behavioural dysregulation.' *Psychol Med* 45(9): 1851–60.

Pistell, P. J., et al. (2010). 'Cognitive impairment following high fat diet consumption is associated with brain inflammation.' *J Neuroimmunol* 219(1-2): 25–32.

Poston, L. (2012). 'Maternal obesity, gestational weight gain and diet as determinants of offspring long term health.' *Best Pract Res Clin Endocrinol Metab* 26(5): 627–39.

Psaltopoulou, T., et al. (2013). 'Mediterranean diet, stroke, cognitive impairment, and depression: A meta-analysis.' *Annals of Neurology* 74(4): 580–91.

Reichelt, A. C. and M. M. Rank (2017). 'The impact of junk foods on the adolescent brain.' *Birth Defects Res* 109(20): 1649–58.

Ruan, Y. et al. (2018). 'Dietary Fat Intake and Risk of Alzheimer's Disease and Dementia: A Meta-Analysis of Cohort Studies.' *Curr Alzheimer Res* 15(9):869–76.

Sanchez-Villegas, A., et al. (2009). 'Association of the mediterranean dietary pattern with the incidence of depression: The seguimiento universidad de navarra/university of navarra follow-up (sun) cohort.' *Archives of General Psychiatry* 66(10): 1090–8.

Sanchez-Villegas, A., et al. (2013). 'Mediterranean dietary pattern and depression: the PREDIMED randomized trial.' *BMC Med* 11: 208.

Schwingshackl, L. and G. Hoffmann (2014). 'Mediterranean dietary pattern, inflammation and endothelial function: a systematic review and meta-analysis of intervention trials.' *Nutr Metab Cardiovasc Dis* 24(9): 929–39.

Shaw, G. M., et al. (2003). 'Neural tube defects associated with maternal periconceptional dietary intake of simple sugars and glycemic index.' *Am J Clin Nutr* 78(5): 972–8.

Simpson, S. J., et al. (2015). 'Putting the balance back in diet.' *Cell* **161**(1): 18–23.

Steenweg-de Graaff, J., et al. (2014). 'Maternal dietary patterns during pregnancy and child internalising and externalising problems. The Generation R Study.' *Clin Nutr* **33**(1): 115–21.

Suez, J., et al. (2014). 'Artificial sweeteners induce glucose intolerance by altering the gut microbiota.' *Nature* **514**(7521): 181–6.

Suren, P., et al. (2014). 'Parental Obesity and Risk of Autism Spectrum Disorder.' *Pediatrics* **133**(5): e1128–38.

Valdearcos, M., et al. (2014). 'Microglia dictate the impact of saturated fat consumption on hypothalamic inflammation and neuronal function.' *Cell Rep* **9**(6): 2124–38.

van Dijk, S. J., et al. (2009). 'A saturated fatty acid-rich diet induces an obesity-linked proinflammatory gene expression profile in adipose tissue of subjects at risk of metabolic syndrome.' *Am J Clin Nutr* **90**(6): 1656–64.

White, C. L., et al. (2009). 'Effects of high fat diet on Morris maze performance, oxidative stress, and inflammation in rats: contributions of maternal diet.' *Neurobiol Dis* **35**(1): 3–13.

Whiteford, H. A., et al. (2013). 'Global burden of disease attributable to mental and substance use disorders: findings from the Global Burden of Disease Study 2010.' *Lancet* **382**(9904): 1575–86.

Whiteley, P., et al. (2010). 'The ScanBrit randomised, controlled, single-blind study of a gluten- and casein-free dietary intervention for children with autism spectrum disorders.' *Nutr Neurosci* **13**(2): 87–100.

World Gastroenterology Organisation, Global Guidelines: Diet and the Gut (2018), http://www.worldgastroenterology.org.

Index